Psychiatric Examination

of Children

Psychiatric Examination of Children

JAMES E. SIMMONS, M.D.

*Professor and Coordinator of Child
Psychiatry Services,
Indiana University School of Medicine*

Second Edition

Lea & Febiger   *Philadelphia* • *1974*

This project was supported in part by United States Public Health Service Training Grant MH 7833.

Library of Congress Cataloging in Publication Data

Simmons, James E
   Psychiatric examination of children.

   Bibliography: p.
   1.   Child psychiatry.   2.   Interviewing in psychiatry.
I.   Title.   [DNLM: 1.   Interview, Psychological—In infancy
and childhood.   WS350 S611p 1974]
RJ499.S56   1974   618.9′28′9075   74-7368
ISBN 0-8121-0494-3

First Edition, 1969

Published in Great Britain by Henry Kimpton Publishers, London

PRINTED IN THE UNITED STATES OF AMERICA

PREFACE

The response to the first edition of this book has been most gratifying. Teachers and students have reported that it does provide, as intended, fundamental technical information around which a student may profitably organize the instructions from his preceptors. Basic examination techniques have not changed in the past four years. Hence, much of the material from the first edition is repeated here. We have greatly expanded the section on the examination of the preschool child with particular emphasis on identifying and treating early developmental deviations. Reality dictates that increasing efforts must continue to be devoted to primary and secondary prevention. Early detection of developmental problems in the very young child must be included in any preventive program along with genetics, family-social environment, reproduction and other considerations.

The difficult task of applying the available scientific nomenclature in clinical practice was omitted from the first edition. In this new edition DSM II of the APA is accepted as our current official diagnostic manual with the hope that the nomenclature of the GAP Report #62 or some modification of it will become officially adopted in the near future. With case examples instruction is offered for the clinical application of diagnostic labels.

It is hoped that the new chapter on consultations will prove to be a significant addition. Consultation is presented as primarily a triage function by which children can more rapidly receive appropriate and definitive psychiatric care. In addition to serving as a sorting station for the psychiatric casualties among children, the consultant must provide emergency and/or short-term goal-limited therapy.

The main purposes of this book remain: to provide step-by-step instruction in diagnostic techniques and to promote clear thinking and precise communication about the clinical phenomenon we observe.

I am indebted to Dr. Gerald D. Alpern for permitting me to use his symptom severity rating scale and for his helpful suggestions on early drafts of the new material in this text. I wish to thank my secretary, Mrs. Judy Barnard, for her invaluable assistance in manuscript typing, proofreading and indexing.

Indianapolis, Indiana

JAMES E. SIMMONS

PREFACE TO FIRST EDITION

In this monograph, written for psychiatrists, pediatricians, general practitioners and medical students, the main emphasis is on the psychiatric examination process itself. In psychiatry the direct interview of the patient has three uses: history taking, diagnostic observations and psychotherapy. The literature contains discussions of various symptom complexes and therapy techniques,* and separate volumes have been published on the systematic use of formal psychologic testing of children.† There is comparatively little, however, in the literature on the direct mental status examination of a child by the physician. The effective way to teach child psychiatry to the specialist or to students is by the preceptor method. Nevertheless, beginners or those who have only limited training time in the child guidance clinic constantly express the wish for written suggestions on the methods of conducting psychiatric interviews with children. This monograph is designed to provide technical information and a frame of reference around which a student may profitably organize his preceptor experiences.

Chess' text‡ provides a very helpful overview of child development, the course of various symptom complexes, and their treatments, as an introduction for the student. The approach in this book is confined more narrowly to instructions on how to make direct behavioral and psychological

---

*See listings 3, 34, 35, 40, 48, and 57 in the Bibliography.

†See listings 9, 10, 30, 42, 43, 45, 56, 59, 60, 69, 71, and 72 in the Bibliography.

‡Listing 18 in the Bibliography.

observations of a child and how to record such observations in clinically useful terms. Very recently Goodman and Sours,* after surveying many professors and teachers of child psychiatry, have offered a highly readable summary of how child interviewing is being taught in various centers. They illustrate the great difficulties in standardizing diagnostic interviews and trying to systematize our methods of obtaining observational data.

There are definite limits to how far standardization of the psychiatric interview can or should go. Unlike the size of the skull, liver, or spleen, or the sounds of the lungs, and heart, behavior has a much wider range of normal limits, and even when deviations are obviously present, they are much more apt to be transitory. Behavior and ideation are always multidetermined. Observable psychologic phenomena are affected considerably by the immediate environment. In contrast, the size of the liver is not altered by an examiner's mere presence, and it is a simple matter to have one's estimate of liver size confirmed by a colleague. In psychiatry the examining instrument is the physician himself, and the examination for the most part is an interaction between two people. The experienced examiner's knowledge of his own personality as a highly significant variable in this interaction process permits him to comprehend the extent to which the patient's behavior is stimulated or altered by the immediate environment. In describing a patient, the examiner must evaluate and report what he himself introduced in each examination. Finally, the interpretation of any behavior is dependent upon many variables, not the least of which is the psychiatrist's knowledge of the whole spectrum of human behavior and his professional grasp of social, cultural, developmental, and psychopathologic phenomena.

In this monograph I have reviewed my own diagnostic

---

*Listing 31 in the Bibliography.

methods as taught by my teachers and my patients. The material is intended to serve as a base line for future refinement of one aspect of child psychiatry: the diagnostic examination. My intent has been to describe examination procedures and to illustrate the integration of the findings into a diagnostic formulation. The student child psychiatrist must learn examining techniques which will detect pathology in children, and must learn to describe his findings in such a way that a colleague of similar training and background would arrive at essentially the same conclusions from reading his report.

Indianapolis, Indiana   JAMES E. SIMMONS

Acknowledgments

I am indebted to many colleagues, residents, and students who have assisted in these efforts to refine diagnostic techniques and communication skills. The ideas originated from the teachers who guided me through my own anxious years of clinical training.

The patience and expertise of Mr. Kenneth Bussy and the staff of Lea & Febiger in the final editing are most gratefully acknowledged.

J.E.S.

CONTENTS

1. Preparing the Child and Initiating the Interview . .   1
   Mutuality of Anxiety   1
   Simple Reassurance for Lessening of Initial Fear   2
   Coping with Nearly Insurmountable Initial
     Resistance   3
   Direct Instruction of the Child   4
   Separating the Child and His Parents on the
     First Visit   5
   Interrogation versus Nondirection   5
   Physical Examinations by the Psychiatrist   6
   Verbal and Nonverbal (Play) Activities   7
   The Psychiatrist's Initiative   8
   Difficulty in Eliciting Spontaneity   10
   Selecting Clues from Initial Play Activity   10
   Confidentiality and Limit Setting   12
   Initiating Interviews with Hospitalized Children   13
   Summary   14

2. General Interviewing Techniques   16
   Equipment for the Interview Room   16
   Training and Personality of the Psychiatrist   18
   Age and Nature of the Child   20
   Structuring the Interview Situation   24
   Reasons for Coming or Being Brought for the
     Examination   27
   Recreation and Interests   27
   Social, Cultural, and Ethnic Group and the
     Child's Harmony with It   28
   Peer Relationships   28
   Plans for the Future   28
   Family Relationships   29

Additional Discussion of the Presenting Problem 30
General Health (Psychophysiologic Status) 30
Fantasies and Fears 31
Social Awareness 32
Summary 32

3. The Mental Status Report 34
   Outline for Mental Status Examination of a Child 35
   Appearance 36
   Mood or Affect 36
   Orientation and Perception 37
   Coping Mechanisms 38
   Neuromuscular Integration 42
   Thought Processes and Verbalization 42
   Fantasy 43
   Superego 46
   Concept of Self 46
   Summary 47

4. Examination of Preschool Children 49
   Communication and Comprehension Problems.. 49
   Special Approaches for Preschool Children 50
   Early Developmental Deviations 67
   Congenital Deformities and Developmental
      Deviations 69
   Summary 77

5. Mental Status Profiles, Normal and Abnormal 79
   Three Preschool Boys 79
   Mental Status Examinations 80
   Pete, Age 2 Years, 6 Months 80
   Billy, Age 2 Years, 5 Months 81
   Steven, Age 3 Years, 4 Months 81
   Comparison of the Metal Status of These Three
      Boys 83
   Relation of Mental Status to the Final Diagnostic
      Formulation 86
   Two School-Age Girls 87

Mental Status Examinations 88
  Jane, Age 8 Years, 5 Months 88
  Abby, Age 8 Years, 6 Months 89
  Comparison of the Mental Status of These
    Two Girls 91
  Comparative Summary 95
  Examination of an Adolescent Who Has Been
    under Chronic Stress 99
  Mental Status Examination of Fred, Age 14 Years 100
  Summary 102

6. Nosology and Diagnosis 104
  Diagnostic Classifications and Formulations 104
  Obstacles to Classification 106
  The Diagnostic Formulation 109
  Summary 112

7. Interviewing the Parents 113
  Two Disparate Attitudes 113
  Interviewing versus History-Taking 116
  Outline for Interviewing the Parents 117
  Child's History 118
  Parents' Marital History 120
  Parents' Personal History and Attitudes
    toward Treatment 120
  Summary 122

8. The Case Study 124
  Outline for Case Study 127
  Refusal to Attend School (School Phobia) 129
  Assaultive Behavior in a 7-year-old 148
  School Failure of an 8-year-old 161
  Summary 178

9. Translating the Diagnostic Formulation into a
    Nosological Diagnosis 180
  Why Classify? 181
  DSM-II (1968) 183

GAP #62 (1966) 185
Special Value of GAP Symptom List 187
The Alpern Child and Adolescent Symptom
Severity Rating Scale 187
Classification of a Case in which the
Psychopathology Seems Not Yet Crystallized .. 190
Summary 192

10. Treatment 194
Severity of the Illness 196
Relation of Severity of Illness to Ultimate
Prognosis 198
Summary 200

11. Consultations 202
Three Types of Consultation Services 203
Consultations in Non-medical Settings 204
Relations of Child Psychiatrists with Medical
Colleagues 206
How Can the Child Psychiatrist Consultant Best
Serve His Medical Community? 207
The Consultant in a Pediatric Teaching Hospital 209
The Process of Consultation in a Medical Setting 211
Identifying Cases for Intensive Psychiatric Care 213
Short Term Psychiatric Treatment 214
Psychiatric Treatment in Conjunction with
Medical Management 216
Psychological Treatment by the Consulting
Psychiatrist 221
Summary 225

Epilogue 227

Bibliography 229

Index 235

Chapter 1

PREPARING THE CHILD AND INITIATING
THE INTERVIEW

MUTUALITY OF ANXIETY

AT THE FIRST clinical visit, there is often deep anxiety in the child, his parents, and the examiner. Children and parents naturally may feel anxiety at their first meeting with a psychiatrist. Each of us also felt apprehensive when he first began seeing children as a psychiatrist. No matter how sophisticated in adult psychiatry and medicine the examiner might be, the knowledge that very young children, even one's own, can handle adults in ways which lessen the adult's control of the interchange is disconcerting, to say the least.

Although outwardly calm, the psychiatrist who is new to the child psychiatric clinic must cope with a number of questions running through his mind. Will the staff laugh if the child does not go readily with him? What will the supervisors say if the child will not talk to him or does not like him? What is he supposed to look for? What if the child is completely incomprehensible? How do you tell the difference between sick and well behavior? What is a normal 5- or 10-year-old like? How can a relationship be established if the child is too destructive? What special knowledge and talent allows the rest of the staff to appear so calm?

These and a multitude of other questions cross the mind of every child psychiatrist and pediatrician in the early part of his professional training. To be forewarned is to be forearmed. It is hoped that the following suggestions about the family's anxiety will also allay some of the initial anxiety of the physician.

The child's and parents' anxiety on their first visit may be a reflection of underlying family problems. Nevertheless, much of the manifest anxiety initially seen should be understood and handled as fear of an unknown situation. Knowledge about procedure can attenuate these fears and make them less painful. Therefore, one should not fail to offer the parents simple instructions on how to prepare themselves and their child for the first visit. The exact words used by the parent will depend upon the age of the child and the parent's estimate of the child's ability to comprehend.

Parents are asked *not* to tell the child that he is being taken to a school to see a teacher, to have tests, or to see a nice man who will play with him. If the child is failing in school, this is common knowledge, as is the parents' concern about it. Therefore the child may be told, "We are going to see a doctor to talk about your trouble with schoolwork." If the presenting symptoms are nightmares, fears, or general unhappiness, the parents should have a similar frank discussion of the symptoms to prepare the child for going to the physician. In general, it is hoped that, through open discussion with the child, the parents can avoid stimulating feelings of shame or excessive fear in him.

A mother's questions about preparing her child may reveal her own feelings in a symbolic manner, but it is not necesssary to confront her with an interpretation of her behavior. It seems best during the intake process to deal with the reality factors of the resistance in an educational manner, leaving the less conspicuous and presumably more neurotic resistances to a later time of diagnosis or therapy.

SIMPLE REASSURANCE FOR LESSENING OF INITIAL FEAR

Harry W.'s mother was slow in returning her clinic application. She telephoned to explain that she was a school teacher and asked whether she could return her application without signing the "permission to obtain a school report" section. She was not certain that Harry's need for help was severe enough to justify the stigma he might suffer at school. The usefulness of school reports was explained to her. We added that at times Harry would need to be excused from school and that usually children discuss their clinic visits with their playmates. These factors negate the possibility of keeping the secret. Prejudice about psychiatry and psychiatric patients still exists. This is something with which we will help the family cope and should not delay or cancel the need to have the study done.

If Mrs. W. had persisted, we would have scheduled an appointment without the release forms being signed. The completed application was promptly returned, however. Later, when given the date of their appointment, Mrs. W. asked whether her husband could be excused because of pressing business matters. She was told that the participation of the father is essential and that we would try to arrange another date to suit his schedule. She thought that perhaps he could adjust his schedule, but, if not, she would call and change the appointment. The family arrived at the originally scheduled time.

The experienced reader will understand that such brief telephone conversations tempt one to make some psychologic interpretations about Mrs. W. Perhaps she was reluctant to expose her maternal behavior to criticism from herself, her fellow teachers, or the clinic staff. Perhaps she had an inordinate need to control and dominate her environment. She may have been afraid that some severe psychosis or retardation would be found in the child or that he could not be helped. These and many other possible explanations for Mrs. W.'s behavior can be explored later at the appropriate time during the history taking.

COPING WITH NEARLY INSURMOUNTABLE INITIAL RESISTANCE

An extreme example is the case of Allen T., age 15. Allen's parents made an urgent call stating that Allen had become violently angry and refused to keep his second appointment with the doctor. He swore at his parents and had begun smashing furniture. They had fled from the house and were calling from the corner drugstore. Mr. T. wondered whether it would not be best for just him and his wife to come to the appointment without Allen. They were asked whether they believed that Allen was homicidal or would do physical harm to them. They were certain that he would not harm anyone, but when he got upset like this they just could not handle him. They were instructed to return home and insist that Allen come for his appointment. If they could not obtain his cooperation, they should call the Juvenile Aid Division of the Police Department. It would be necessary for them to file a complaint in order that the boy might be placed in the Juvenile Detention Home. Once this placement was effected, arrangements could be made with the authorities to complete our examination of Allen. In about 30 minutes the parents appeared at the office with an angry but compliant Allen. The police had not been called. It took several visits to complete the study, but it was eventually possible to establish a working relationship with Allen.

Such strong-arm tactics should be the exception and used only as a last resort. Coercion or other forms of force are not favored, but they may be necessary if the child may possibly do some irreparable harm to himself or others. One might argue that an emergency psychiatric hospital should be used for such cases. Patients, however, cannot wait for adequate or "ideal" facilities to be built. It is possible to do a complete psychiatric evaluation on a youngster who is under legal detention, provided the psychiatrist has good working relationships with the local authorities and is willing to put up with some inconvenience to himself.

DIRECT INSTRUCTION OF THE CHILD

Whether preliminary interviews with the parents, telephone advice, or coercive measures have been used, most children come for their first visit without understanding the purpose of the examination. The child may have been too anxious, antagonistic, or distrustful to believe or even hear the parents' explanation. On the other hand, the parents may have been so anxious about the visit that they could not even approach the subject and have just brought him in, saying nothing or having given him only half-truths and evasions. Therefore some preparation of the child on the first visit by the psychiatrist is essential. (For details of how the author instructs the child, see page 8.)

SEPARATING THE CHILD AND HIS PARENTS ON THE FIRST VISIT

In our clinic we usually meet the child for the first time with his parents in the family group intake session.[70] The staff and the family engage in open discussion of the family's concerns and of the clinic's procedures. During this group meeting the child is told that he will have some sessions alone with specific examiners.

The ease with which the child separates from his parents has some diagnostic value. Difficult separation may be owing to a pathologic tie between parents and child or to the child's anxiety in response to new situations and new people. It should be noted, however, that difficulties in separating the child from his parents can also be inversely proportional to the experience and comfort of the examiner. If the examiner is afraid or expects that he will have trouble, he frequently does.

Since it is not possible to know immediately the significance of the clinging behavior, it is best not to make this separation forcefully. There is certainly no harm in permitting one parent to accompany you to the playroom, with the instruction that he or she may return to the waiting room as soon as the child is reassured. On rare occasions, for either the mother's or the child's comfort, or both, it is necessary for a parent to remain throughout the interview session. By action and by words, however, the examiner should indicate that on subsequent interviews he will try to make this separation. In a few cases, this separation has actually been part of the treatment for both mother and child. Usually, by the second visit, separation should not be a problem.

INTERROGATION VERSUS NONDIRECTION

Planned use of the physician's time is extremely important. It is necessary for him to be friendly, relaxed, and unhurried. If he assumes the role of an authoritarian interrogator, such as may be seen in some law enforcement agencies, he produces uncooperativeness, negativism, and relatively few data. On the other hand, the examiner cannot afford aimless, rambling, nondirective chitchat which usually reveals little about the child.

Interview sessions should be limited from 30 to 60 minutes for the convenience of the examiners' own schedule, as well as to avoid fatiguing the child. At our center, students are expected to see a child at least twice and preferably three or four times for a psychiatric examination, with a time interval between visits. No matter how experienced the examiner is, an advantage of at least a second interview is that anxiety due solely to the newness of the situation will be less. More important is the fact that it takes time to know a person, and it is rarely possible to do a complete mental status evaluation in less than two or three interviews.

PHYSICAL EXAMINATIONS BY THE PSYCHIATRIST

The doing or requesting of a "routine" physical examination merely to rule out organic disease is useless, because ruling things in or out is a never-ending responsibility. Nevertheless, before visiting the psychiatric clinic, all children should be seen by their family physician or pediatrician, because it is essential for every child to have a physician who is fully responsible for his organic well-being and for the commonly accepted prophylactic measures against illness.

A physician's report outlining organic illnesses should be part of the child's psychiatric case record. Beyond that, medical judgment should determine the need for requests for physical or neurologic consultations. From the history or during the course of observation, the psychiatrist may raise questions about specific aspects of the child's physical health. Appropriate questions are then resolved by the psychiatrist's own further investigations, with the aid of consultants. A consultant can always give an expert opinion on a specific question but is as impotent as anyone else in definitively ruling out organic factors.

In a medically isolated location it may be necessary for the psychiatrist to serve as his own neurologic consultant and do whatever procedures are necessary to answer questions raised about the child's physical status. Ekstein[23] takes the opposite position, feeling that physical examinations should never be done by one who is or intends to become the child's psychotherapist. In our opinion, the child psychiatrist need not abdicate the responsibility inherent in his medical background. He must raise questions about possible organicity and work with his medical colleagues to find answers to these questions. This kind of responsibility begins when the patient enters the clinic or hospital and ends only when he is completely discharged.

VERBAL AND NONVERBAL (PLAY) ACTIVITIES

In our clinic we prefer to use a combined office-playroom setting for interviews. This provides a greater flexibility and permits the child to accept either the conversational or play type of interview, or a combination of both. Its secondary advantage is that each person may keep his work space as neat or messy as he chooses, and the administration does not have to deal with the constant query, "Who left the playroom in a shambles?"

The psychiatrist's activities are designed to make the child as naturally spontaneous and cooperative as possible. The author usually tries the conversational method of interview even with very young children. Nondirective free play should not be relied upon exclusively. Lack of interview structure can make some children more anxious, because they think that the examiner is avoiding the real purpose of the visit. Other children may quickly learn to use play as a means of indefinitely avoiding talking to the physician.

In either fantasy play or in direct discussion, the examiner should encourage the child to take the initiative. Do not be so passive as to create a new anxiety in the child but, so far as possible, allow him to initiate and direct the play. A suitable balance between play activity and direct conversation comes with experience. The activity-passivity ratio varies considerably among equally competent psychiatrists and will also vary according to the examiner's estimate of what approach will be productive with a given child.

Many novice examiners, without realizing it, enter a playroom with a child and immediately go to the doll house (if they are with a girl) or pick up the guns (if with a boy). By this action the examiner initiates play, and the child will then reflect the examiner's fantasies rather than produce his own. Adults seem to have an uncontrollable need to engage in some activity when they are with children. The obvious toys in the room are usually invitation enough, though you might add, "This is my room. You may use any of the things here." (If you use a combined office-playroom, you cannot have personal things on display which you would not permit the child to use.) The stated question, "What would you like to do?" is out of place. The psychiatric interview is not a den meeting or a summer camp where children must constantly be doing something to satisfy their leaders.

THE PSYCHIATRIST'S INITIATIVE

If the child does not take the initiative, it often helps to discuss quickly with him the reason for his clinic visit. This is the examiner's obligation and his opportunity to prepare the child for interviews. The child should be asked what he was told about coming and then asked for his fantasies, thoughts, and guesses about coming. If he can give any information, he is asked how the actual experience compares with what he was told or what he imagined about the event.

If he does not know or was not told, he may be asked to guess why others might come to the clinic. If the child responds with any statements at all, it is then possible to correct any erroneous ideas he may have and allay his anxiety. If he comes up with nothing, he may be told that the examiner is a doctor who helps people with their troubles or worries and problems. Children come to see him because of worries or problems about their friends, their family, their school, or themselves. If the child does not pick up these suggestions, he can be told that his parents were worried because he does not sleep well, because he is unhappy at home, or because things are not going well for him at school, whichever is the case for him. With delinquent children who are highly suspicious, it is frequently useful to say that we understand they are in detention or have been in some trouble and would like to hear their side of the story.

If the patient cannot or will not use such openings to talk about the presenting complaints or other topics, it is useless to push questions or conversation in the initial interview. More important, the child should understand you are not an object to be feared. You are definitely interested in him as a person, and you at least know of the existence of his problems. Mentioning problems early may be useful only to try to dispel the suspense about what the examiner knows.

Often the entire first interview is spent trying to put the child at ease and clarifying the purpose of the visits. With some children, anxiety and confusion about the examination are not problems, and one can proceed to obtain as much of the data outlined in the next sections as time permits. The psychiatrist should remember that the amount of data he obtains will often be inversely proportional to the amount of pushing or authoritarianism used.

The reader may feel that this admonition against pushing a child too authoritatively is contradicted by the previous illustration of Allen T. Allen's case was unusual, however, and was used to illustrate extreme action which is only *rarely* necessary in order to do a thorough examination. Allen was a very angry and uncooperative boy, and our threat to use police action to control his behavior did not endear us to him. On the other hand, he did not become violent or mute, but excused the examiner for his (the examiner's) behavior on the grounds that we did not understand what he had "to put up with" around the house. He spontaneously reassured us that he would not actually harm "them," even though he felt like it at times. He caustically suggested that we had forced him to come in order to be certain that we collected our fee for the time. Even though he doubted our abilities and our intentions, the situation at home was so bad that he thought he would keep subsequent appointments to see what we could do.

DIFFICULTY IN ELICITING SPONTANEITY

Marilyn, age 8½, was brought to the clinic because of a severe school phobia. She separated from her mother without difficulty but in the playroom sat with a "frozen" body posture. Tears were in her eyes, but she did not cry. Her pupils were dilated, her hands trembled, and her speech was a barely audible whisper. Attempts to discuss the scary feelings of her first visit did not produce any relief, nor did invitations to play with toys. After 15 minutes she did accept an invitation to go down the hall for a Coke. She drank it slowly and looked at the pictures on the wall around the building. Her body posture relaxed, but she remained too tense to talk or play. On the way home she told her mother that she was "really scared, but the doctor bought me a Coke and it made me feel better."

Sometimes it is impossible to relieve a child's fear of the examination except through gradual lessening of the anxiety with each succeeding visit.

SELECTING CLUES FROM INITIAL PLAY ACTIVITY

Permitting the child to take the initiative in the interview produces valuable material. Often the child may begin by telling you in words or action some symbolic illustration of his presenting problem, his feeling about the examination, or both.

John, age 7½, was referred for aggressive behavior at home and at school. He rushed to the playroom the instant he was invited. He quickly took the guns and shot wildly around the room with vivid sound effects and descriptive phrases such as

"I got 'em! He's dead! You dirty Jap!" He tried to shoot the examiner but was easily persuaded to direct his fire at the targets and the doll figures. As the intensity of his play subsided, he began to talk about his father and of the fun they had fishing, boat riding, and playing ball together last summer.

In this instance it was not necessary for the psychiatrist to become active or take the initiative; indeed, such was probably contraindicated. John appeared acutely anxious and demonstrated that he handles anxiety by overactivity. He further showed that his behavior can be controlled by mild prohibitions when he acquiesced to the request to shoot inanimate targets rather than the examiner. He also evidenced inner control by gradually stopping the aggressive play. This is in contrast to some children, whose aggressive actions tend to snowball in intensity and will cease only with strong external prohibitions.

The diagnostician needs to learn to identify the feelings revealed by play and the sources of these feelings. Violent shooting can be a direct expression of angry feelings and possibly a defensive cover-up for strong fear. In John's case it seemed highly probable that both fear and anger were stimulated by the examiner and the clinic visit. Had John been asked directly to describe his feelings about coming to the clinic, he might have confirmed this hypothesis.

The fact that John's violent play subsided so easily with a willingness and a desire to talk about his father made the examiner feel that factors outside the clinic experience were more related to John's behavior. Usually the examiner would have some history that would provide additional clues to the meaning of the behavior. In this instance the history was not available until after the initial interview. (Such a procedure should be done occasionally to sharpen interviewing skills.)

John's spontaneous, glowing account of his positive relationship with his father made the examiner suspect some problem with the father. It is usually safe to pursue any topic introduced by the patient. Therefore John was asked to tell more about his activities with his father. When asked about things which caused disagreements and conflicts between him and his father, John revealed that his father had died six months ago. Without a strong emotional display, plans for the summer recreation that never took place were reviewed.

John was a highly active boy whose aggressive feelings spilled out but were brought under control easily. His father had died recently, and John was still struggling with the mourning process. His desire to shoot "dirty Japs" and the physician, followed by a glorification of the father relationship, was a graphic portrayal of ambivalence to the lost father. Child psychiatrists frequently find that strongly emotional and significant topics determine the initial play activity in the first interview. Equally often, the child may avoid these same topics for several weeks in subsequent interviews.

> An 11-year-old delinquent boy opened the interview by bragging about how much he liked to have his immunization shots. He spontaneously told about a doctor friend back home who permitted him to go on house calls and sometimes give the shots. Sensing his fear, the examiner volunteered that he would not be given any shots. The patient responded by saying he had thought that the examiner would give him a blood test. The examiner explained that he wished to talk to the boy about the troubles he had been having. The patient responded that there were some things he would not care to discuss. He then launched into a long discussion of legal procedures followed by a detailed account of the inner workings of automobiles.

This boy was not a car thief. Rather the entire first interview was concerned with his fear and distrust of the physician and probably all adults. He also revealed that he had developed some skill in the arts of evasion and prevarication as a means of handling threatening adults.

CONFIDENTIALITY AND LIMIT SETTING

Limit setting and confidentiality are issues which the examiner must keep in mind during the initial interview and in all subsequent interviews during both diagnosis and therapy. The limits that will be set or enforced and the degree to which the psychiatrist can be trusted are problematic to the relationship.

On the basis of experience the child does not readily trust adults, especially strangers. If you are trustworthy, the child will come to trust you. With some children, however, this will not occur until treatment is completed. When a child stares at our note-taking or looks for hidden microphones, we should try to get him to discuss his concern for confidentiality. One cannot swear to absolute and eternal secrecy about the interviews, but one can promise the youngster that he will be told when we plan to talk with his parents or others and will be told in advance what we will tell them.

Limit setting is such a personal matter, charged with the professional's attitudes and feelings about aggression, that it cannot be dealt with adequately on the printed page. The effect of limits on the productivity of an interview is probably dependent upon both the conscious and unconscious intent of the examiner, his timing, and his intuitive grasp of the child's need for permissiveness or limits, as well as the past experience and nature of the child's illness. If you consistently have unproductive hours, you may be too restrictive. On the other hand, if the playroom is always a shambles and the patient is in an agitated state after your interviews, you may be either failing to set limits or unwittingly stimulating the child to act out. In either of these instances, some firsthand observations of your interviewing techniques by a colleague or supervisor would be much more helpful than a printed discourse on limit setting.

INITIATING INTERVIEWS WITH HOSPITALIZED CHILDREN

The psychiatrist's introduction of himself to a child hospitalized on a general medical ward requires a different approach from that described for the initial outpatient visit. Hospitalization can be frightening in itself, and being taken to strange places in the hospital can provoke unnecessary anxiety if the child is unprepared. It helps to have the psychiatrist visit the child first at his bedside and introduce himself. Has the attending physician explained the purpose of the consultation? If not, an explanation and the reason for the referral should be given to the child in much the same way as instructions are given to the parents for preparing the child. The term "psychiatrist" is well known to many children, but it is best not to use this term until the child indicates some comprehension of the psychiatrist's function. One can make a comparison between his own role and that of the attending physician. "We are both doctors. However, while Dr. Jones examines your sore throat, or your tummy, or your chest, I'm a doctor who is particularly interested in children who have problems, worries, or troubles. I do not plan to undress you or listen to your heart, since that has already been done, but Dr. Jones would like me to talk with you about some of your problems."

Usually the children's ward presents many stimuli about which one could talk for a few minutes. Some inquiry should be made about how long the child has been there and how he feels about it. If there is sufficient privacy from the other children, he may briefly discuss his problems. It is our practice then to inform him of our plan for a playroom or office interview. He is told the time and place of the interview and given some instruction about the location of the office in relation to his own ward.

It is not possible to cite all potential variations of the initial interview. The majority of introductory sessions with patients go smoothly, and fortunately, patients are usually charitable about our blunders. Nevertheless the initial interview is troublesome to the patient, to the novice examiner, and in some instances it may adversely affect all future attempts to work with the patient. Hence the physician can well afford introspective evaluation of his initial interviews.

SUMMARY

The initial interview for examination usually provokes anxiety in both the child and his parents. This experience also heightens the discomfort of the examiner when he first begins his study and practice of child psychiatry. Advance instruction of the parents for preparing themselves and the child, and simple reassurance, will usually lessen much of the initial fear. It is also important sometime early in the interview for the psychiatrist to offer the child some explanation of clinical procedures and reassure him about his knowledge of the child's problems.

Occasionally, initial resistance and anxiety may be nearly insurmountable. It is important for the physician to recognize that the anxiety accompanying the first visit may unduly influence the child's behavior and that one must be cautious about drawing hasty conclusions from the initial interview. Although a firm stand or even force may occasionally be indicated with a particularly rebellious child, a patient, easygoing approach is usually more successful than authoritative questioning.

It is the author's conviction that physical examinations or consultations, when definitely indicated, are the responsibility of the examining physician and will not unduly interfere with the establishment of a relationship if thoughtfully and properly performed.

Eliciting spontaneity in the child can be difficult. There must be an opportunity for both verbal and nonverbal activities during the interview situation. The examiner must avoid being so passive that he frightens the child unduly, but at the same time he must permit the child free rein for fantasies with as little direction and suggestion as possible.

Some illustrations for selecting clues from the child's play activity are presented. Confidentiality should be assured by both words and deeds of the examiner. The matter of limit setting during the interview situation will vary greatly, depending upon the personality and tolerance level of the examiner. Yet if the psychiatrist is too restrictive or if he fails to offer the child any behavioral guidelines, the child's productivity in the interview may be seriously distorted.

Chapter 2

GENERAL INTERVIEWING TECHNIQUES

THE INFORMATION to be obtained during the child's examination is the same as that needed for the mental status examination of adults: e.g., orientation, affect, stream of thought, fantasies, ambitions, concept of self, interpersonal relations, ideals, mannerisms, and so on. The methods of obtaining these data depend very much upon the age and nature of the child, the training and personality of the examiner, and the setting in which the examination takes place. The psychiatric examination is incomplete until sufficient material is obtained to write a complete mental status report. This is time-consuming and will take several interviews.

EQUIPMENT FOR THE INTERVIEW ROOM

In general, a greater number of possible activities are needed for ongoing psychotherapy than for diagnostic interviews. A wide variety of activities, as well as the opportunity to do things and to do them together with the therapist, are often essential in therapy. In our clinic we maintain two traditional playrooms which any staff member may schedule for specific hours when use of his own office-playroom might be impractical.

The following items may be found in either or both of these rooms: pullman kitchenette for cooking and baking; sinks for water play; space for large-muscle activities; a variety of art materials such as clay, paints, and crayons; tools and woodworking bench; building blocks; baby dolls; miniature-life dolls; puppets; toy soldiers and guns; furnished doll house; assorted trains, trucks, cars, and planes; sandbox; models for assembly; and assorted table games. The exact content of the rooms varies somewhat from time to time, depending upon the fads or convictions of the staff. So far as possible, most of these materials are kept in cupboards with sliding doors to facilitate periodic cleaning of the room and to give the therapist some control over the amount and kind of stimuli presented to a particular child.

It may be impractical for the lone practitioner to maintain such a variety of equipment for a comparatively smaller number of patients. Although the items noted are often, but not always, needed for continuing child psychotherapy, we have found the following quite adequate for diagnostic interviews and much of our therapy in the playroom-office combination: some creative art materials, some toys for aggressive fantasy play, a few action toys (trucks or cars), dolls or puppets for depicting interaction and personal projection, and some table games to be used for interaction with the examiner and to permit evasion of or relief from emotion-laden activities.

Besides the playroom and adequately equipped offices, the child psychiatrist finds many other readily available settings he can use. Children's general distaste for close confinement and the fact that they are less inhibited about personal matters than adults make it permissible to take young patients out of the playroom or office at times. The elevator and the basement of a building are most interesting and stimulating. The street, the local playground, the drugstore soda fountain, the construction projects in the next block, and many other areas can be considered part of the child psychiatrist's interviewing equipment.

The decision to take a child outside the office or playroom has its pitfalls. Most people learn at a very early age that discomfort in social situations is relieved by either changing the subject of conversation or by moving about, preferably to a different setting. If the examiner becomes anxious for any one of a variety of reasons, he may take the child "out to play" to "help him relate better." Psychiatrists are so accustomed to talking about such things as sex, violence, or sadness that we don't feel uncomfortable with the verbal child, no matter what he says. However, symbolic play of these emotions, refusal to say or do anything, or gestures and words which are too personally directed may provoke us to take the child out of the examining room without realizing it is our own and not the child's discomfort which is being handled. A decision or action by the examiner is correct if it facilitates the purpose of the hour. Sometimes we cannot be sure about the correct action until we have tried it. When a child is taken out for play during a diagnostic exam, we must ask ourselves if we learned anything about the child. If not, then we would have done well to have remained in the office. We tread a narrow line here. It would be cruel to confine a child to the office if he is overwhelmed with his own thoughts and fears. On the other hand we do the child no favor if we engage him in activities which prevent him from ever revealing himself.

TRAINING AND PERSONALITY OF THE PSYCHIATRIST

The formal training requirements and examination procedures necessary to obtain recognition as a specialist in child psychiatry are outlined by the Subcommittee on Child Psychiatry of the American Board of Psychiatry and Neurology, Inc.[5] These include fulfillment of all the training and licensing requirements for general medical practice, training and certification in general psychiatry, and finally special training and examination in child psychiatry. Hence from a pragmatic standpoint the kind of person who becomes a child psychiatrist is predetermined by various admissions officers or the admissions committees of colleges, medical schools, general psychiatric residency training programs, child psychiatry training programs, the American Board of Psychiatry and Neurology, and that organization's Subcommittee on Child Psychiatry.*

---

*From the mid-1940's until the formation of the American Board subcommittee on Child Psychiatry, 1959, training standards were formulated and monitored by the American Association of Psychiatric Clinics for Children.

Finally, a local medical society, a state medical licensing board, the board of directors of a community clinic, and parents will have some say in determining the sort of person who will be the psychiatrist for any particular child.

Whether or not the long, arduous, and rather cumbersome selection process which has evolved really provides us with those persons from the total population who are best suited to fulfill a specific mental health need for the next generation may be debated — in fact, is rather hotly debated at times in some circles. It can be said with certainty that each selecting authority numerically reduces the field of choice for the next higher authority. No doubt some persons are kept out of the profession who would have much to offer, while others with comparatively little potential slip through this screening network. We can only hope that the numbers in each of these categories are small. If so, this is indeed fortuitous, since few of these selecting bodies have the specific selection of someone to care for mentally ill children as their primary concern.

Every young man or woman who considers entering the profession should give serious thoughts to his own suitability. He is aware that interest and motivation are primary factors that have many unconscious determinants. These and other unconscious elements of his own personality may serve him well or poorly in his future work with children. The fact that children, especially sick ones, create an emotional impact upon the adult makes it essential that the child psychiatrist have considerable insight into his own behavior. In addition to helping the resident trainee accumulate knowledge and clinical skills, a major goal of many, perhaps most, preceptors is to help the resident develop useful insight into his own emotional responses to his patients.

In the past, many preceptors insisted upon personal psychoanalysis for their child psychiatry candidates as a means of providing this insight. Even though some still hold to this tenet, it has appeared to many as neither entirely practical nor at times particularly effective. One might say the same for child psychiatrists as can be said for parents: for many, personal psychotherapy is essential to reach even a modicum of success as either a parent or a child therapist; for others, effective functioning can be greatly enhanced by therapy. Certainly the matter deserves serious consideration by each trainee and his supervisors. At this time, however, no absolute rules about personal analysis seem possible. The child psychiatrists of this country serve in a variety of functions — as therapists, diagnosticians, researchers, administrators, and child care consultants, to name a few. No one can ever be the epitome of perfection in all these areas. The candidate should use his own conscience and the observations of his preceptors to determine whether his daily work is socially and professionally effective and, if not, to determine whether therapy for himself is the answer.

Preparation for work in child psychoanalysis is beyond the scope of this monograph. The interested reader may be directed to sources of information regarding training in child psychoanalysis by the American Psychoanalytic Association or by a psychoanalytic institute in his geographical area.

AGE AND NATURE OF THE CHILD

Of the three variables in the diagnostic interview — the examination setting, the examiner himself, and the patient — the most important is the patient. It would take many volumes to discuss each age level and the many behavioral variations related to age. Here, however, a few general comments about children as psychiatric patients are in order.

There is great danger of skewing all the information if one is preoccupied too early with delineating normal and abnormal behavior. The assessment of normality or abnormality is discussed in the next section. During the examination itself, the emphasis should be upon learning to know the child as thoroughly as possible without jumping to conclusions or making value judgments.

Great allowances must be made for children's attitudes toward the examiner and the examination. Many children appear resistive and negative when brought to the psychiatrist's office. From the child's standpoint these attitudes are completely justified. The child psychiatric patient is similar to the committed adult patient in that usually he had no part in the decision to seek professional help and has been brought for the examination against his will. His past experience may well have proved that all adults are in collusion, and he feels that the examiner is no exception. Certainly he knows that there was some communication between the examiner and his parents in order to arrange the appointment "behind his back," and since his parents are paying the fee it is only natural that the psychiatrist's alliance would be with them. He believes that adults really have little interest in understanding children except for nefarious purposes. Commonly, whether the child admits it or not, he firmly believes that the examination will give positive proof of his innate badness and will justify further punishment from his parents.

A language barrier can present problems between the physician and his patient. Adolescents and certain ethnic groups often use colloquialisms and dialects in a conscious attempt to maintain their privacy from the conventional world. Younger children are still developing from primary process thinking to secondary process thinking. Their ability to use abstract concepts and to express feelings and ideas at a verbal level is often limited. These limitations provide one reason why play is so essential to child diagnosis and therapy. The child can express himself in action much more easily than with words.

Adults usually have considerable difficulty in comprehending the play language of children. The chapter in Erikson's book[24] entitled "Toys and Reasons" is strongly recommended to the student of child psychiatry. Erikson reminds us that, to the adult, play means recreation or respite from work. On the other hand, play is a principal occupation of childhood and has much more personal significance than merely a relief from the workaday world. Play activity usually has a common meaning for a group of children of similar age and background. It will also have a unique meaning for any individual within the group. To comprehend the unique meaning, one must not only observe the play's content and form but also have the child tell his accompanying fantasies and reveal the affect associated with the play. Erikson believes that much of the unique meaning of play is concerned with the child's efforts to master himself, his own body and body sensations, and the anxiety stimulated by the world and events around him. Through play the child learns to master reality by experiment and planning. Erikson points out that it is a definite human trait at any age to deal with experience by creating model situations. He quotes William Blake: "The child's toys and the old man's reasons are the fruit of the two seasons."

For obvious reasons the dissocial or delinquent child can be expected to be considerably more resistant to the examination than the average child. Aichhorn[2] explains that these children, particularly those lacking in neurotic guilt over their behavior, approach all adults with a negative transference of distrust and hostility. The adult must be able to take the child's part and agree with his behavior under the circumstances. When these children boldly lie or maintain stoic silence, the examiner should control his irritation and the usual adult impulse to expose the culprit's hostility and untruthfulness. Sometimes distrust can be attacked directly by agreeing that it is dangerous to confide in strange adults but reminding the patient that some subjects can be mutually discussed without this danger. Aichhorn lets the child know that he is not fooled by him, but neither is he angry over these justifiable attempts at trickery. To make this point he sometimes uses gentle, transparent sarcasm in the form of spoofing the child by telling grosser lies.

Frank, nonjudgmental discussion of the child's delinquent actions can disarm him and help him to confide to you his concept of the outer limits of right and wrong. No matter how far he is from the social average, each individual has some line or point beyond which he considers behavior to be wrong. Some homely examples are the common belief that it is all right to steal small amounts, but not large ones, or that it is not particularly reprehensible to pilfer from the government or large corporations, but it is serious to appropriate a neighbor's possessions. The following case illustrates the use of frank, open discussion as a means of ascertaining the standards that have been internalized by the patient.

Jack, an 11-year-old, had been placed in juvenile detention for stealing and vandalism, and his court worker had requested a psychiatric evaluation. After a brief general conversation, the subject of his detention came up. Jack quickly professed his innocence and the fact that he was implicated by others on purely circumstantial evidence.

Examiner: I know that, but tell me—under ordinary circumstances what do you like to steal the most?

Jack: Oh, anything, just anything.

E: What's the most you've ever really been able to get away with?

J: Oh, I guess a bicycle worth about twenty bucks. Oh, yeah, I got fifteen dollars from my uncle Harry's dresser once.

E: See my fountain pen. Would you steal that?

J: No, not unless I was sure I could get a running start on you.

E: How come they claim it's always wrong to steal from banks and stores when those places got lots of money?

J: Cause you will get sent to prison for it.

(This last comment portrays reliance upon external controls as a major deterrent to antisocial behavior.)

After some additional conversation on other topics, the matter of sex was approached. Jack volunteered that he knew everything about that.

E: How old were you when you first had sex with a girl?

J: It was last year when I was ten.

E: Was she your girl friend?

J: Nah, she was my cousin.

E: What happened?
J: My aunt caught us.
E: What happened?
J: She told my mother.
E: What happened?
J: My mother said you ain't supposed to
do that with your relations.

It is essential to remember that the psychiatrist is not assigned the task of extracting a confession. His task is to obtain a professional opinion of the over-all functioning of the patient. Therefore, questions are not designed to learn whether or not an act has been committed. One may ask questions as if the fact of their occurrence had already been settled. The child is then free to deny the implied allegations, or he may decide that, since guilt or innocence is not an issue, he can readily reveal the details. Some delinquents will enjoy responding to the question, "How did you happen to get caught?" but are made angry by questions about why or whether a certain act was committed.

STRUCTURING THE INTERVIEW SITUATION

Werkman,[73] Beiser,[12] Martin,[50] and many others have described their interview approaches, which are varying combinations of play and conversation. Manipulating the child's play according to some memorized structured interview procedure is apt to suppress the child's spontaneity. On the other hand, mere passive observations of the child's play without eliciting any verbal associations may leave the examiner confused as to the specific significance of the child's activities.

This author uses a moderately active conversational method of interview in an office-playroom. In general, children under 10 or 11 years of age are most comfortable and productive when using the play materials, while older children readily respond to the conversational method of examination. Some 14- or 15-year-olds, however, spontaneously use the toys, usually as a tension-relieving device. On the other hand, some 6- or 7-year-olds, unable to use the play materials, are able to indulge in direct conversation about themselves and the significant events or people in their lives.

As stated previously, children should not be encouraged to "do" something or be forced to play. If they appear interested, they can be told that they may use any of the things in the room. If they play spontaneously, questions may be interjected from time to time to clarify the action and thinking. If they seem content to sit and talk, let them do so. Should they become increasingly anxious in the examination instead of more spontaneous, they may be taken out for a walk or a treat or urged to play.

There should be an abundance of time for any interview. The examiner's activity-passivity ratio must be geared to a level that will promote the child's productivity, and his approach will have to be altered considerably from child to child. The patient should be given ample opportunity to be spontaneous, keeping in mind that prolonged silences can be anxiety-provoking to many children. On one occasion after a one-way-vision room demonstration, a group of medical students asked whether the examiner was purposely using silence to provoke and upset the patient. The examiner had not been aware that the patient was particularly anxious. Whether the child was unduly distressed by the silence or not remains uncertain, but the medical students had reacted negatively to it. It has been our observation that medical students push and talk too much in interviews. Psychiatrists are apt to err on the side of overusing silence.

The word "why" should be avoided as much as possible. "Why?" often sounds too much like an accusation or implies that the situation is wrong and needs justification. If the child knew the answer, he probably would not need professional help. Children have been negatively conditioned by adult use of the word "why." Often a parent asks, "Why did you do it?" or "Why didn't you do such and such?" During a play situation the question, "Why did doll 'A' run out of the house?" may disrupt the play. Putting the question as, "What was doll 'A' thinking about when he ran out of the house?" may facilitate the child's associations. Asking the patient why he or she wishes to be a fireman or policeman or a nurse when he grows up implies that he must justify his decision. It is better to ask what policemen or nurses do that he finds particularly interesting or fun. Instead of asking why a particular event in his history occurred, he can be asked, "Where were you and what were all the people doing just before that happened? How were you feeling? How did it make you feel afterwards?" The following is a list of ten broad, general topics around which an interview may be loosely structured.

1. Reasons for coming or being brought for the examination
2. Recreation and interests
3. Social, cultural, and ethnic group and the child's harmony with it
4. Peer relationships
5. Plans for the future
6. Family relationships
7. Additional discussion of the presenting problem
8. General health (psychophysiologic status)
9. Fantasies and fears
10. Social awareness

As mentioned previously, the child will often initiate the interview by acting out his problem or illustrating something significant in his interpersonal relations. He may talk directly about these subjects or use symbols and play. During the course of several interviews, some children will spontaneously give considerable information on each of the foregoing topics. Others will spontaneously include most of the items, and with relatively few questions the examiner can obtain information on subjects which did not come up spontaneously. Still other children will require a considerable amount of activity on the part of the examiner.

The topics may be covered in any order that seems natural. Frequently it helps to ask questions indirectly or buffer them with comments such as, "Some kids have told me they expected the clinic to be a lot different than it is." "A little girl [boy] told me the other day that she had lots of trouble with her brothers and sisters. Have you ever known anyone who felt like that?" Teachers, playmates, or parents may be substituted in that question for brothers and sisters. Whenever possible, the open-end type of question is used. If questions meet with silence, the child is permitted to remain silent or pursue other activities.

Reasons for Coming or Being Brought for the Examination

Ask what the child has been told and what he thought the purpose was. Inquire about his feelings about the visit. If he has been told nothing or does not know, suggest that he guess, or that he guess why others might come to see the physician. He can be reassured if he expresses fear about the visit. The examiner should identify himself and his reasons for interest in the child. If you know that there is particularly severe antagonism between the child and his parents, it is occasionally helpful to reveal this knowledge to the child and invite him to tell his side of the story. This approach and these questions were discussed in the section on the initial interview. However, when the child is unwilling to discuss his problems, it is useless to try to probe deeply until you are comfortable together, possibly not until the second or third interview.

Recreation and Interests

When the child spontaneously reveals some of his special talents or interests, it is an easy matter to gain considerable information by polite questions about details. If he gives you no clues, he can be asked directly about his hobbies or the kinds of things he thinks are particularly fun. The interview is helped by talking about nonproblem areas or areas of success, and considerable information about the child's abilities and interests or lack of them, compared with his age group, can be learned. On these topics one should be able to see a child at his best and note his organization of thinking, his stream of thought, his attention span, and perhaps even obtain clues to his intellectual capabilities.

Social, Cultural, and Ethnic Group and the Child's Harmony with It

Inquiries may be made about school, church, and the neighborhood. What things does he like best about these places, and what does he like least? What are the people like whom he finds there? What do his parents say about these places? Ask what is most troublesome in school: the teachers, the studies, or the other children? Has he ever changed schools, or would he like to? What kinds of things are or would be different at the other school?

Peer Relationships

Knowledge of peer relationships as the child sees them will give considerable information about his capacity to make meaningful interhuman relations, his identifications, his degree of social awareness, and his level of independence. Does he have one friend or a few best friends, or does he claim social relations with nearly everyone? What are the depth and nature of these close relationships, if they exist? Do they tell each other secrets? How frequently are they in contact? What kinds of things do they do together, and how do they settle their disagreements? Who are some of the kids he doesn't like or who do not like him? What kind of differences do they have? Inquiries about clubs and team memberships are appropriate, and the child should be encouraged to compare himself with others in his age group as to relative size, intelligence, leadership, and so on.

Plans for the Future

When asked what they would like to be when they grow up, most children appear embarrassed and say that they do not know yet. They can be reassured that you know the final decision cannot be made at this time. Yet almost all of us think of a number of things from time to time that we would like to be, even though we change our minds. What are some of the things that he has considered? What do people of that vocation do? Which of these activities has any special appeal? Some little girls say that it would be fun to be a nurse because she helps sick children, while others believe that it would be fun because nurses get to give shots. Some children see a policeman as maintaining law and order, while others admire him as someone who has legal sanction to shoot people.

After growing up and finding his work, does the child think that he will marry? Has the potential partner already been chosen? What does he think he would like best about being married, and what least? Would he like to have children of his own? How many? Would he rather have boys or girls, and what are the relative advantages? What has he been told about where babies come from and how they got there?

Family Relationships

The child should be encouraged to tell about the pleasant family relationships and the fun they have both as a group and individually with siblings, as well as with the mother and father separately. He could then be asked about what kinds of things might make them angry with each other. How do the family members express their anger, and with whom are they most often angry? When someone is angry, how does the patient and how do the parents react to this? How much does the child know about his parents' vocations, and how does he feel about their work?

Very young patients may be presented with a simple drawing of a mother and a child which the examiner has sketched. The drawing should be neutral about the child's sex. The patient is then asked to describe what he sees. He will usually give the child the same sex as his own. He can then be asked the age of the child and about relations between mother and child. He can be asked what the child does to make his mother happy or angry and what the mother does when she experiences these feelings. What kinds of things does the mother do that make the child particularly happy or angry? What does the child do when he experiences these feelings? The same sketch may be used, substituting a father for the mother.

Additional Discussion of the Presenting Problem

Even though the child may have been willing to discuss the presenting symptoms during the initial phases of the first interview, it is always a good idea to review problem areas directly with him in some detail after the relationship has been established. He can be asked whether they seem to be getting worse or better and how worried about them he might be. Ask what he thinks might help. Inquiry can be made about previous examiners or therapists, if there have been any, and his concept of how the examiner might help him or his family with their difficulties.

General Health (Psychophysiologic Status)

Psychophysiologic difficulties can be ascertained by inquiry into past sicknesses or injuries and the patient's reaction to these events. If he has not volunteered the information, he should be asked about current somatic symptoms; when appropriate, a menstrual history can be taken. Questions about eating habits, sleeping habits, and general physical well-being can be postulated. If one suspects poor contact with reality, inquiry can be made about visual or auditory difficulties, and the child can be asked about any visions or voices.

> On one occasion when the author was examining a 12-year-old boy who appeared to be responding to voices, inquiry was made about his general health and whether he had any hearing difficulties in the form of buzzing or sounds or speech that others did not seem to hear. The boy turned to the examiner and replied, "I beg your pardon, Doctor, but I do not have hallucinations."

The child may be asked to draw a person and then a person of the opposite sex and sign his name. If he will tell stories about his figures, these will increase the examiner's knowledge of the child's self concept and his interpersonal relations. At the very least, drawings will give some grasp of the child's fine motor coordination. The drawings may be used to score a rough estimate of the child's intelligence following the Goodenough Draw-A-Person Test.[30] Silver[66] has reviewed Goodenough's test and has added some ideas of his own on the diagnostic value of children's drawings of persons.

Fantasies and Fears

Much of the content of the interview may be the patient's fantasies. Any story he will tell or any game he will make up is part of his fantasy, as are his freehand drawings or paintings. None of these fantasy productions is distinctively characteristic of any specific condition, but each can give impressions about the child's contact with reality, his intelligence, the predominant feelings he has, his concept of himself, and his degree of inhibition or lack of inhibition as to feelings. If the child will verbally associate and will display feelings in relation to his fantasy productions, the unique meaning of his play will be revealed. Often his play will reflect family relationships or past experiences.

In addition to his spontaneous productions, one can inquire about his nicest dreams, his scariest dreams, and any repetitive dreams. One can ask for his earliest memory and for three wishes; they may often be associated with his deepest psychologic problems. One can offer him the possibility of three money bags, with which he may do anything, as a substitute for the question about three wishes.

Inquiry about fears and worries can be made directly from any clues the child may have given. Often the child will feel that he is the only one with such fears or worries, and one may offer him reassurance. He can be asked his ideas about what happens to people who die and about any fears he might have about dying.

Some additional clues about his identification and his most problematic feelings can be learned by asking what kind of animal he would like to be and what particularly appeals to him about that animal.

Social Awareness

Often, by directly or indirectly inquiring about the limits of the playroom situation, the child will reveal something of his concept of right and wrong or his concern about possible loss of control. Occasionally the child may be asked directly whether he thinks certain things are right or wrong and why he thinks so. Questions about social activities and interests will already have revealed a considerable amount about the social-cultural standards of the child's background. Matters of social control and limits, as well as a sense of right and wrong, may well be emotion-laden topics, the child already having had considerable experience with the differences between the adult's world view and his own view of these matters. Hence any questions that must be asked should be framed in a nonjudgmental and fact-gathering manner.

SUMMARY

Interviewing techniques depend upon three variables: the child, the examiner, and the examination setting. The setting may be a playroom or office, but the author prefers a combination of both. Equipment should facilitate the child's verbal and physical expressions. He may be taken out of the office or building to facilitate the establishment of the relationship. In the office there should be opportunities to talk or play. The availability of a wide variety of toys and creative materials helps the child freely express his fantasies. Fantasies become clinically meaningful to the examiner when the child verbalizes his accompanying thoughts and the associated affect is noted.

Child psychiatrists need to recognize that their own emotions are significant factors affecting both diagnostic and therapeutic work. No absolute rule can be made about whether all child psychiatrists should or should not have a personal psychoanalysis or psychotherapy as an essential part of training. Certainly a definite goal of the training should be the development of insight into any aspect of the psychiatrist's personality which might impair his effectiveness with his patients. Whether analysis or personal therapy is essential for the candidate's training is a matter which he must decide for himself in consultation with his supervisors.

In general, children are highly resistive to psychiatric exploration and therapy. It is essential to recognize the reality basis of much of the resistance. This is particularly true for delinquent children. Negativism and resistance to the psychiatrist's efforts to relate to him can be lessened somewhat by having the utmost patience, using the open-end question whenever possible, being open and aboveboard at all times, and making every effort to avoid being or appearing judgmental.

Ten broad, general topics around which the author loosely structures interviews have been listed. Considerable detail about the child in each of these reference areas is needed. Examples of the kind and amount of detail needed are offered in the discussion. It is hoped that the child will spontaneously and freely reveal this information. When he does not, exploratory questions or activities which stimulate the child to reveal himself should be used.

Chapter 3

THE MENTAL STATUS REPORT

CHAPTERS 1 and 2 concentrated on techniques for interviewing children. This section will present an outline which we have found useful for organizing and recording the observations of the clinical interviews. The student physician must learn to gather clinical data and write up his findings in a manner which is comprehensible and useful to himself and his colleagues. The psychiatrist's account of his firsthand observations of the patient constitutes the mental status report.

To facilitate professional communications and to increase objectivity and accuracy, it is essential to have a set of factors which can be regularly examined and systematically recorded for each child. Such a set of factors must be items available for examination in a wide variety of children, definable with reasonable clarity, and capable of depicting qualitative and quantitative variations. In our practice we have used a modification of Beres'[13] systematic evaluation of ego functions of schizophrenic children. The observable aspects of the child's personality constitute his ego and the conscious part of his superego. These personality facets are present with variations in every child, whether he is severely disturbed or relatively healthy.

The categories presented here are not the only possible subheadings that can be used for a mental status report. When properly defined, however, ego functions have provided us a good descriptive frame of reference. Terms such as "ego strength" and "ego adequacy" are not sufficient. The ego is not a "thing" but a group of related and overlapping functions.

Freud[28] described the ego as a functional part of the personality "entrusted with important functions." For our thesis it is not relevant to discuss how the ego functions develop. Rather, we intend to list a group of psychic phenomena which by common usage have come to be regarded as ego functions.

The mental status report is a description of the child's appearance and behavior during two or three hours of psychiatric interviews. If the ego functions outlined below are carefully examined, it is likely that neither significant pathology nor personality strengths will be overlooked. The diagnosis can be vague and confusing if significant ego deviations are overlooked and not recorded or if only deviant aspects of the personality are noted, overlooking the more or less intact ego functions.

The listing of these items for the mental status report is not intended as a regimentation of interviewing. It merely serves as a standard guide for recording the kinds of observations needed. Not all the items can be considered ego functions. Each, however, is either an ego function or reflects upon one or more ego functions. Ego functions do not separate distinctly like the movement of the right arm and of the left arm. Therefore the division of these items has been rather arbitrary, as has also the order of their listing.

OUTLINE FOR MENTAL STATUS EXAMINATION OF A CHILD

1. Appearance

2. Mood or Affect

3. Orientation and Perception

4. Coping Mechanisms
   a. Major defenses
   b. Expression and control of sexual and aggressive impulses

5. Neuromuscular Integration

6. Thought Processes and Verbalization

7. Fantasy
   a. Dreams
   b. Drawings
   c. Wishes
   d. Play
8. Superego
   a. Ego ideals and values
   b. Integration into personality
9. Concept of Self
   a. Object relations
   b. Identifications
10. Awareness of Problems
11. Intelligence Quotient Estimate
12. Summary of Mental Status Evaluation

Appearance

Appearance can give clues to ego functions, such as identifications that the child seems to be making, his need for conformity or nonconformity to various social groups, and his socioeconomic subculture. It is not enough to state that a child is dressed appropriately or inappropriately for his age and social group, since only your best friends will know what you mean and they may disagree with you. Some children are ardent conformists to nonconformist groups. Therefore, a description of the child's size, appearance, and manner of dress should be written as part of the mental status. Such things as severe acne, obesity, and obvious handicaps should be noted as either possible causes or results of chronic emotional problems. Mannerisms, tics, and speech disturbances should always be recorded descriptively.

Mood or Affect

Mood or affect refers to the predominant feelings displayed by the patient. How does the mood fluctuate or change during the interview, from interview to interview or from topic to topic? Is the youngster able to demonstrate the full range of affects? For instance, a child may look flat or frightened in the beginning, but as he relaxes he may reveal that other feelings dominate his consciousness even more. The ease or lack of ease with which a child handles and displays different emotions is helpful in diagnostic assessments.

Orientation and Perception

These ego functions reflect much about the child's ability to see and comprehend reality. In assessing the child's orientation we are comparing his intellectual grasp of reality to his age and social peer group's knowledge of time, place, and person. Perception refers to the kinds of impressions he gains about things or events by the use of his special senses.

In assessing perception we need to know to what extent he clearly differentiates fact from fantasy. By the age of 3 or 4 some ability to differentiate should be evident, and by 6 or 7 years a healthy child can make clear distinctions between his fantasy life and his reality situation.

In addition to clarifying with him which events are make-believe, we can ask him to tell about his clinic experience. If he was not told about the clinic, what kind of guesses does he make? Can he recount his trip to the clinic? Does he recognize the toys? Can he figure out the use of a new toy he has never seen before? Does he respond to visual and auditory stimuli outside the room? Does he respond to the stimuli inside the room? Naturally, it is necessary to know that the perceptual mechanisms for sight, hearing, smell, touch, and so on are organically intact.

Irrespective of the age of the child, it is important to observe which of his senses—sight, hearing, touch, and taste—he uses. By noting the qualitative and quantitative use of these senses and using our clinical judgment, we can ascertain the age appropriateness of his perceptive abilities. For example, it is age-appropriate for a 5-year-old to examine a variety of toys and objects in a room, using all the special senses, before selecting something which interests him. A 15-year-old would more appropriately explore the room with his eyes only and for a briefer time. Seriously disturbed children of any age vary from a constricted use of the sense organs to an extreme of hyperperceptiveness wherein minor stimuli appear to intrude themselves forcefully into consciousness.

Orientation is the patient's knowledge of objects and persons, including himself, and their relations in time and space Does he know his name, address, birth date, seasons of the year, parent's occupation, and where he is? A true mental concept of time in terms of hours, weeks, and months is often not very clear to the child until about the age of 8 or 9. We need to know how far he has progressed in learning time relations and concepts. We can discern this by discussing events in his personal history and daily life and by noting his ability to understand time between clinic visits. When told that his next visit will be a week from today, at two o'clock, a 5- or 6-year-old may ask whether he will see you tomorrow, but such a question would be inappropriate for a 9- or 10-year-old.

Coping Mechanisms

Coping mechanisms are the ways in which the patient handles strong emotions, instinctual impulses, and nonspecific anxiety. What defense mechanisms does he try to use? Which defense mechanisms predominate in the interview? In other words, does he act out, deny, avoid, rationalize, intellectualize, project? Unfortunately, clinicians do not have absolute agreement on the precise definition of the defense mechanism terms. Even so, we must pay particular attention to the child's coping methods and mechanisms in our interviews. To avoid confusion, a verbal description of the child's behavior is recorded, omitting the use of psychologic jargon or reserving the use of terms to brief conclusions in the summary. The following examples illustrate this.

The body of a mental status report contained a direct observation in which Harold, age 11-years, claimed he knew all about babies. When pressed to tell what he knew he seemed startled and confused but then quickly replied, "Oh, yes, that's the one where your father starts out, 'Now, son, I've noticed you're at the age when you should know certain things —' I know all about babies. I don't want to talk about that stuff any more."

Referring back to this observation, the summary of the report contained the following: "Discussion of sexual matters provoked anxiety in Harold which he tried to handle intellectually but then could only handle by evading and avoiding the subject."

"Intellectualization," "evasion," and "avoidance" are healthy defense mechanisms if not used excessively. The actual clinical significance of this boy's reactions can be assessed only in relation to the total case work-up and cannot be considered *a priori* evidence of a serious sexual problem. The introduction of the topic of sex did produce obvious anxiety, as it does in most children of this age.

The point to be made here is that accurately recorded mental status examinations can be used to assess changes in the patient which occur over periods of time. If only the summary had been recorded, it would have been impossible to assess qualitative changes in the child's knowledge and reactions about sex unless all subsequent examinations were done by the original examiner who had an infallible memory.

Diversions of the course of play or conversation constitute a form of coping used by patients of all ages. When this phenomenon occurs, the examiner may assume that the child is trying consciously or unconsciously to cope with anxiety. Is the source of the anxiety: the situation of coming to the physician, something about the physician himself, the subject matter of the play, or a high degree of anxiety related to deeper problems which plague the child no matter what the subject or setting?

Space will not permit a comprehensive list of the innumerable varieties of coping mechanisms used by individual children. We assume that every person has sexual and aggressive impulses which must be handled at the ego level. Everyone also has anxiety from a variety of other sources and will function in certain ways which he has learned will keep the anxiety at the lowest possible level for him. We are therefore interested in how successful his coping mechanisms are (a) in relieving his feelings of anxiety and (b) for facilitating his individual functioning. Note the contrast in the following two cases:

> Betsy, age 7½, silently took the examiner's hand and went to the playroom. She did not speak or look at the examiner. Her facial expression was blank. After only a momentary glance around the room she crawled under the play table, pulled her knees up to her chest, and closed her eyes. She did not move when the examiner touched her. Her pulse and breathing were slow and steady.

> Billy, age 8, appeared inordinately frightened but would look at the examiner and whisper brief answers to questions. The examiner tried to talk to him about the scary feelings children often have when they go to the doctor. He said that this was all news to him and that he had never had any of those feelings. His pupils were widely dilated, and his breathing was rapid. Since talking did not relieve him, the examiner invited him to use the playroom facilities and materials. Billy merely sat and squirmed in the chair. The examiner's silence seemed to make him even more anxious. The examiner then took the initiative to divert him into a game. Billy complied with instructions but never relaxed. When the time was up, he could not get down the hall fast enough. None of the things he used and none of the things the examiner used had been completely successful in relieving the anxiety.

One may speculate that Betsy was overwhelmed by anxiety. Contrariwise, one could also speculate that she was free of conscious anxiety since she did not show any of the usual physical concomitants of anxiety. Even if we conclude that her withdrawal successfully relieved her of a conscious feeling of anxiety, we must also conclude that her methods of coping with the situation were such that her total functioning was seriously impaired.

Billy showed a high degree of anxiety which he was unable to relieve and which affected his ability to relate to the examiner and to use the toy room for his own pleasure. His anxiety was greatly relieved by the termination of the interview, but he did not totally withdraw from the examiner until given permission to do so.

The behavior of both children was so significantly different from that of the average child that we felt safe in concluding that their reactions were not solely in response to the immediate environment. Although both children used avoidance and withdrawal, Billy's behavior more nearly approximated the psychosocial behavior of his age group. Additional interviews with both children spaced at intervals of several days or a week were indicated to explore other areas of their functioning and to learn whether familiarity with the examiner and his surroundings would lessen the anxiety response to the clinic visits themselves.

Billy's behavior changed only slightly in two subsequent diagnostic interviews. On the basis of history and other findings it was concluded that he was suffering a severe neurotic adjustment reaction brought on by an extremely traumatic home situation, and a trial of weekly therapy sessions with him and his parents on an outpatient basis was instituted. As he relaxed during the ensuing weeks and months, the physical signs of anxiety disappeared. He became able to use the toys in structured games and finally became able to indulge in fantasy play and conversation with his therapist.

Betsy's behavior had been essentially as described for several months. She was hospitalized for further study. It seemed that some of her sleepiness might have been an untoward response to previous tranquilizing medication. Discontinuation of all medication did result in a wider variety of behavior, but communication with others by touch, gesture, or eye contact remained minimal, and she never spoke more than a few unintelligible words in a singsong manner. While both of these children could be said to be manifesting avoidance and denial, on qualitative assessment Betsy is by far the sicker of the two.

Neuromuscular Integration

We need to know the degree of activity of the child and to observe his gross and fine movements. How does he handle a ball? Can he handle the mechanical toys? Are his movements smooth or jerky? Very young children, some psychotic children, some infantilized children, and some brain-damaged children show varying degrees of difficulty with motility and coordination.

Thought Processes and Verbalization

Information about the child's spontaneous speech and verbalization is often available as soon as you meet him. We also include his play as part of his spontaneous thinking.

> Dr. Z reported a "frustrating" interview with Christopher. "I didn't learn a thing because he just wouldn't talk to me." The supervisor asked what the child had done. "Well, he just sat there and drew. He wouldn't look at me or talk to me. He drew a house, and then there were some figures put on the house, and then he wouldn't discuss the drawing. Then he scribbled over it with black crayon."

Chris' home situation had an abundance of severe problems. Even though silent with the examiner, he failed to hide the fact that he was preoccupied with a home and the people in it. Play is thinking, albeit partly unconscious.

We are interested in the rate, sequence, form, and quality of the thinking and in any special preoccupations the child has. Often certain themes recur in spontaneous play or conversations which give clues to problem areas. As clinicians we are interested in problems and the child's view of his symptoms. Yet, as noted in a previous section, children seldom, if ever, have a part in the decision to seek help, and it is not surprising that most children cannot or will not discuss "problems." Indeed, we always consider ourselves fortunate if a child will engage in spontaneous conversation about any topic of interest to him. Just letting him talk will give much information about his vocabulary, his sociocultural milieu, his interests, his relationships, his ability to relate, and his ability to organize his thinking.

Fantasy

In the outline at the beginning of this chapter, we included dreams, drawings, wishes, and much of the play activity as subdivisions of fantasy. Fantasy is a part of the thinking processes. It is also a reflection of other ego functions. Sometimes fantasy is used as a major coping mechanism. The child's fantasies also can reveal much about his perceptive and intellectual abilities. Fantasy play or stories usually reveal problematic areas in the child's intrapsychic and interpersonal experiences. Quantitative and qualitative aspects of fantasy production are important diagnostically. Yet neither fantasy nor any other single part of the mental status evaluation can be considered conclusive or pathognomonic of any specific condition.

From clinical experience we know that the severely hedonistic, relaxed, glib, acting-out child usually displays a dearth of fantasy material. He does not remember or is unwilling to tell his dreams. His wishes are either for concrete, material objects of great value or are exaggeratedly altruistic. "I can't think of three wishes. The only one is that there never be any more wars and everyone everywhere will always be happy" was the pious wish expressed by one 11-year-old whose history was replete with antisocial acting-out behavior. He engaged in no fantasy play and was evasive and brief when the examiner attempted to engage him in storytelling. Although his wish seemed to be presented as a conscious effort to tell the examiner what a nice, good boy he is, it also implied a wish to alter or abolish the violent aggression and resultant unhappiness in himself and his world.

There may also be a low quantity of fantasy material in highly anxious, extremely inhibited, neurotic and schizoid children. In these cases the verbal inhibitions are not so selective as with the acting-out child. At the opposite extreme, some acutely schizophrenic children may show that fantasy dominates most of their waking hours, nearly excluding reality considerations.

Qualitatively, fantasies which deal with real life problems indicate a reasonably healthy use of fantasy as a coping device in both healthy and moderately neurotic children. Such phenomena are seen in children who use doll play to act out, perhaps ventilate, their experiences of visits to the physician or the dentist, a hospitalization, or the loss of a loved pet or playmate. Fantasies replete with sadism, sexually symbolic behavior, and megalomanic world destruction, with little or no relevance to the child's reality situation, are seen in borderline psychotic and severely neurotic children. Overtly schizophrenic children who permit adults to learn their fantasies are apt to reveal undifferentiated sexual-aggressive ideas of bizarre content with tangential and dissociated themes. The impression is a flood of confused, garbled thoughts.

Whether the fantasies are revealed through free play, drawing, dreams, or wishes, it is always important for the examiner to assess the child's ability to distinguish fantasy from reality. Students frequently complain that supervisors stretch their imaginations to make something significant out of the child's play. After all, dreams are dreams and play is play. Students often ask, "Since all children indulge in fantasy, how can you tell normal from abnormal fantasies?"

The question discloses the medical students' wish to oversimplify diagnosis by easily and sharply separating normal and pathologic phenomena. Except for extremely bizarre, violent, or overtly sexual fantasy play or verbalizations, the content often does not reveal either pathology or normalcy. It is usually not possible to answer the question of "How pathological?" on the basis of content alone. We are interested in whether a child *uses* fantasy in a healthy or unhealthy way and whether he can distinguish it from reality. More importantly, we want to know the child's thoughts and feelings. Fantasy permits a child to reveal his thoughts and feelings to an adult more comfortably than does direct conversation. He may not know that he is talking about himself as he makes up play or tells a story. Should he suddenly realize that he is revealing intimate thoughts, or should his thoughts frighten him, he can always relieve the attending anxiety by reminding the examiner that it is all "make-believe."

It is common practice to ask for the child's three wishes. Sometimes he wishes for something which will obviously change a problematic situation, such as, "I wish my mother and daddy wouldn't be divorced any more." Often the child's wishes are merely popular, common ones. Like the popular Rorschach responses, they do not give clues to problem areas. Common wishes do indicate, however, that some of the child's thinking is in tune with that of his peer group. "Affectionless" and dependency-deprived children do not talk about needing love and security. They are apt to wish for food, money, or lavish material possessions. Often inquiry into what a child would do if the wish were granted will produce clarifying fantasies.

Much of the same can be said about dreams. Many children enjoy telling their scariest, nicest, most recent, or repetitive dreams. Children cannot free-associate to their dreams, and this is probably not desirable, since the examiner always treads a narrow path between learning as much as he can and yet avoiding the stimulation of overwhelming anxiety. Nevertheless, the more details a child will give about his dreams, the more one learns about the thoughts he has when the conscious censor or guard is asleep at the gate.

It goes almost without saying that free play not only helps to put the child at ease with the adult examiner but also reveals his emotional expressions and his thoughts about himself and the world around him. Drawings and the child's discussions of his productions are useful in the same ways. (See page 31 for the use of drawings in a more standardized way as diagnostic aids.)[30,66]

Much more research needs to be done if drawings or

spontaneous fantasies of any form are to become standardized projective techniques. The child's free play and fantasies offer such a rich source of information about him as a person on an empirical basis that one questions whether further standardization of this material is necessary, desirable, or even possible.

Superego

We can observe or examine only the conscious part of the superego. We are interested in the child's ideals and his value system. To what extent does his concept of good and bad or right and wrong seem to influence his behavior? Does he seem preoccupied with antisocial or forbidden impulses? If so, is the result an excessive constriction of behavior or an opposite lack of control? When there is lack of control, either the impulse to act out is inordinately strong or the child is totally dependent upon the external environment to set limits for him because internalization has not occurred. Sometimes these children have identified with antisocial adults and have internalized a corrupt superego. The constricted child may also suffer pressure from strong impulses to act out. He, however, has either incorporated a rigid superego or his fear of loss of control and inability to judge acceptable limits make "no action" the only possible mode of behavior.

Naturally, it is important to know his intellectual concept of right and wrong. Beyond that we should try to learn the discrepancies between stated standards and actual, internalized standards. Is his superego a source of frequent or constant anxiety, or is it an automatic regulator of behavior which helps avoid anxiety-producing situations and thus actually facilitates his social interactions?

Concept of Self

We put concept of self, object relations, and identification in a group together because these aspects of the ego seem intimately related and do not permit a separate discussion or examination. It seems to be splitting hairs to try to make distinct categories out of each of these. For instance, the child's concept of himself is closely tied to his identifications and to the kinds of relations he has established with other people.

Beres[13] states that the child develops from narcissism to true object relations, from inadequate self-awareness to self-identity, from transient identifications to the permanent identifications which lead to ego and superego formation. The immature human being goes from confusion of identity to a definitive sexual identity. The development of all these aspects is in active, dynamic flux in the child, subject to progression and regression according to the various inner and outer forces acting on him at any given time. Diagnostically, we are interested in the qualitative and quantitative aspects of the self concept, the object relations, and the identifications as the child reveals them at the time of the examination. The central issue of determining whether there is retardation of development or regression from a more developed state must rely on accurate history and often on prolonged observation for an answer.

Does the child see himself as strong or weak, good or bad, large or small, handsome or ugly, and in comparison with whom? How does he approach and interact with the examiner? From direct observation, from his play, and from his conversation, how would one describe the feelings which predominate his daily negotiations with his parents and siblings? What are the number and the depth of his friendships? How does he characterize the people in the world?

The last three items on the list—awareness of problems, intelligence quotient estimate, and summary of the mental status evaluation—are not ego functions. They do not need special definition and will not be discussed further.

SUMMARY

The child psychiatrist must be able to comprehend his patients as distinct, functioning individuals. His comprehension of the patient is tested by his ability to write down diagnosis and for communication with colleagues. We have offered a list of ego functions as a moderately standardized frame of reference for describing a child as he is seen during examination. It is our thesis that diagnosis will be improved if the physician concentrates on describing both the assets and the liabilities of the personality. He must control his urges to delineate sharply the "pathologic" from the "normal" until he understands the person and has at least a historical overview of his life situation.

Our experience has been that the use of this list of ego functions as a mental status examination outline promotes depth and thoroughness of examination by our student psychiatrists. It has the additional advantage of providing a graphic account of the child which can be used for comparison later.

The mental status report is a cross-sectional word picture of the child at a given time, under special circumstances. The clinical significance of these findings will increase in value as they are related to the child's sociofamilial situation and past history. The outline for case study and the case summaries in subsequent chapters illustrate the integration of the mental status report with other clinical data.

Chapter 4

EXAMINATION OF PRESCHOOL CHILDREN

IT IS COMMONLY thought that preschool children are particularly difficult to examine psychiatrically because of their limited verbal ability. Our own experience has been that the vast majority of preschool patients, even as young as 2 years of age, are quite capable of verbal interchange with adults if given enough time. It is also possible to learn a great deal about a child by observing his interaction with others, his use of toys, and his manipulation of his own body. Consequently, our approach with these children is essentially the same as described in Chapter 2, with appropriate modifications for the examiner's handling of the interview process.

Under ordinary circumstances, 2 or 3 hours of free play with a preschool child will provide the examiner with sufficient observational data to draw a few conclusions about each subdivision of the mental status examination outline discussed in Chapter 3. One's own observations can be amplified by the history from the parents. Some examiners spend little or no time directly examining preschool children and rely too heavily upon parental observations. There is a great danger in this practice. Parents are naturally not objective about their own child and their reports may erroneously minimize or exaggerate the child's functioning abilities and disabilities.

COMMUNICATION AND COMPREHENSION PROBLEMS

It is a pleasure to watch the ease with which two or three preschool children can interact and communicate. Most of us had excellent ability to communicate with 3-year-olds when we were also in our preschool years. Unfortunately, in the process of becoming an adult, social conditioning, repression, suppression and intellectualization seem to have become highly developed at the expense of our ability to enjoy social interchange with very young children. Some grown-ups do not talk *with* youngsters. They appear to talk *at* them or talk down to them in a patronizing way. Others, especially men, appear to be most ill-at-ease in relating to infants and toddlers in any way except the authoritarian role. One is tempted to speculate that our culture conditions the male to reject prolonged or intimate contacts with the very young. Such a generalization has many exceptions. However, the ease with which a "grandfather type" communicates with preschoolers is often impressive. Perhaps he is less preoccupied with worldly matters and has more time than younger men. It is equally possible that by the grandfather age men are no longer afraid to display talents which society says inherently belong to females. During high school and college many women gain experience with infants as baby sitters and mother helpers. Comparatively few young men have this background.

Whatever the reasons are, it does seem that child psytrists in training and many with years of experience are very unsure of themselves when asked to examine or treat preschool children. Fortunately, this situation is changing and an increasing number are devoting a major proportion of their professional energies to the study of preschoolers. Some training centers offer didactic instruction and supervised experience in well-baby clinics and nursery schools. In addition, the training child psychiatrist should seek every opportunity among his family and friends to care for and play with infants and toddlers. Not until one has learned to maintain his composure in the presence of runny noses, dirty pants and screaming wigglers can he be comfortable enough to objectively observe infantile behavior.

SPECIAL APPROACHES FOR PRESCHOOL CHILDREN

Even when the examiner is completely relaxed, some preschool children may be particularly difficult to examine if extreme fearfulness or some profound mental disturbance constricts their play or interferes with their verbal and nonverbal communication. The author is indebted to Dr. Marian K. DeMyer[21] for permission to publish verbatim the following examination outline designed by her. In her work with several hundred pre-school children over the last twenty years, Dr. DeMyer developed a series of eight "maneuvers" to facilitate the interview process and to help objectify the observational data. Her work reported here represents one of her early attempts in the development of a structured psychiatric examination for research purposes. However, we feel her approach is equally applicable to ordinary clinical practices and should not be limited to research investigations.

Maneuver #1

Examiner goes into observation room where child is with parent(s). Examiner introduces self to parent and child: "Hello, Mr. and Mrs. ————. Hello, (Name of child) ————. I'm Doctor ————."

RESPONSE OF CHILD

Affective Reaction
( ) No change in expression
( ) Cries
( ) Tears
( ) Screams
( ) Smiles
( ) Laughs
( ) Frowns
( ) Bland, neutral expression
( ) Fear
( ) Anger

Reaction to Parent(s)
( ) Goes to parent
( ) Talks to parent
( ) Looks at parent
( ) Ignores parent
( ) Parent soothes child who:
    ( ) Kicks or hits
    ( ) Clings to parent
    ( ) Pulls away
    ( ) Continues crying
    ( ) No obvious reaction
    ( ) Talks to parent
( ) Child in physical contact with parent when E. enters room

Reaction to Examiner
( ) No obvious reaction
( ) Goes to E.
( ) Looks at E.

( ) No eye contact
( ) Average eye contact
( ) Above-average eye contact
( ) Moves away from E.
( ) Moves toward E.

REMARKS:

Maneuver #2

Examiner walks to child, extends hand to child, tries to look at child's eyes, and says, "There are some toys in my office. Let's go play with them."

RESPONSE OF CHILD

Affective Reaction
( ) No change in expression
( ) Cries
( ) Tears
( ) Screams
( ) Smiles
( ) Laughs
( ) Frowns
( ) Bland, neutral expression
( ) Fear
( ) Anger

Reaction to Examiner
( ) No obvious reaction
( ) Moves away from E.
( ) Runs or paces around room
( ) Manipulates body
( ) Manipulates toys
( ) Moves toward E.
   ( ) Assaults
   ( ) Takes E.'s hand
( ) Pats hand
( ) Other reaction to E.'s hand
   Remarks:

Reaction to Parent(s)
( ) Goes to parent
( ) Talks to parent
( ) Looks at parent
( ) Ignores parent
( ) Says goodbye
( ) Waves goodbye
( ) Parent soothes child who:
   ( ) Clings
   ( ) Continues crying
   ( ) Stops crying
   ( ) Talks to parent
   ( ) Pulls away
   ( ) No obvious reaction
( ) Child in physical contact with parent when E. enters room

Reaction to Examiner (con't.)
( ) Converses
( ) Above-average eye contact
( ) Average eye contact
( ) Below-average eye contact
( ) No eye contact
( ) Resists leaving room
( ) Has to be carried
( ) Leaves easily
( ) Makes verbal plea to E. to stay with parent

Maneuver #3

In Examiner's office, E. says to child, "You may play with any toys you like." E. sits on chair three or four feet away from child and watches child's activities for 7 minutes. E. talks to child only if child initiates conversation. E. does not ask questions and replies as briefly as possble to child's questions or conversational attempts.

Toys Used	Touches	Mouths	Describe Repetitious Use	Describe Appropriate Use	Combines	Imaginative
Ball						
Blocks						
Cow						
Cowboy hat						
Doll						
Doll bath						
Doll blanket						
Doll bottle						
Doll clothes						
Golf club						
Gun and holster						
Horse						
Indian headdress						
Lawn mower						
Musical bear						
Musical book						
Puppet						
Rake						
Refrigerator						
Rifle						
Stove						
Sweeper						
Tinker Toys						
Tommy gun						
Top						
Train						
Wind-up bear						
Another object						

RESPONSE OF CHILD

Affective Reaction
( ) No change in expression
( ) Cries
( ) Tears
( ) Screams
( ) Smiles
( ) Laughs
( ) Frowns
( ) Bland, neutral expression
( ) Fear
( ) Anger

Verbal Reaction
( ) Initiates conversation
( ) Talks to toys
( ) Talks to self
( ) Echolalia
( ) Reversal of pronouns
( ) Babbling
( ) Noises
( ) Mostly silent
( ) Sings words
( ) Hums
( ) Words clear
( ) Pronouns appropriate
( ) **Other**
     Describe:

Use of Body
Large mm coordination
     ( ) Good
     ( ) Average
     ( ) Poor
Small mm coordination
     ( ) Good
     ( ) Average
     ( ) Poor
Amount of activity
     ( ) Above average
     ( ) Average
     ( ) Below average
     ( ) Idiosyncratic activity
          Describe:

Response to Examiner
( ) Looks at E. and smiles
( ) Climbs on E.'s lap
( ) Sits close to E.
( ) Stands close to E.
( ) Looks at E. without smiling
( ) Does not come near E. physically
( ) Above-average eye contact
( ) Average eye contact
( ) Below-average eye contact
( ) No eye contact

Maneuver #4

Examiner sits down face to face with child and does the following:

1. Asks: "May I play with you?"

RESPONSE OF CHILD

Affective Reaction

( ) No change in expression
( ) Cries
( ) Tears
( ) Screams
( ) Smiles
( ) Laughs
( ) Frowns
( ) Bland, neutral expression
( ) Fear
( ) Anger

Verbal Reaction

( ) Starts appropriate conversation
( ) Says "yes"
( ) Says "no"
( ) Nods yes
( ) Nods no
( ) Speaks words, phrases, sentences appropriately
( ) Echolalia
( ) Pronoun reversal
( ) Babbling
( ) Noises
( ) Sings
( ) Silent most of time
( ) Other
    Describe:

Use of Body

( ) Remains in same position
( ) Turns or moves away from E.
( ) Touches E.
( ) Sits on E.'s lap
( ) Runs around room
( ) Idiosyncratic activity
    Describe:

Eye Contact

( ) Above-average eye contact
( ) Average eye contact
( ) Below-average eye contact
( ) No eye contact

2. E. talks with child about his activity, then says to child, "We are going to play some games for a while." If child balks at changing activity, E. should do and say whatever will help the child comfortably shift his activity. E. says, "Let's play ball for a while. Get the ball." If child has not fetched the ball himself in response to E.'s suggestion, then E. should get the ball and say, "Let's roll (or toss) the ball to each other." Then roll it on the floor to the 2- and 3-year-olds and toss it gently to the 4-, 5-, 6- and 7-year-olds.

RESPONSE OF CHILD

Affective Reaction

( ) No change in expression
( ) Cries
( ) Tears
( ) Screams
( ) Smiles
( ) Laughs
( ) Frowns
( ) Bland, neutral expression
( ) Fear
( ) Anger

Verbal Reaction

( ) Says, "all right" or equivalent
( ) Says "no" or equivalent
( ) Converses appropriately
( ) Inappropriate verbal response
( ) Echolalia
( ) Pronoun reversal
( ) Babbling
( ) Noises
( ) Sings
( ) Silent most of time
( ) Other
    Describe:

Use of Body and Ball

( ) Gets ball and tosses to E.
( ) Gets ball and keeps
( ) E. has to pick up ball first
( ) Tosses ball to E. 3 or more times
( ) Tosses ball to E. 1 or 2 times
( ) Plays odd or unusual game
( ) Holds ball but won't play
( ) Won't touch ball
( ) Idiosyncratic body activity
    Describe:

Eye Contact

( ) Above-average eye contact
( ) Average eye contact
( ) Below-average eye contact
( ) No eye contact

Attention to Activity

( ) Concentrated in activity
( ) Attention wanders
( ) No attention to activity

( ) Good coordination
( ) Fair coordination
( ) Poor coordinaton

3. With graduated, multicolored ring set, E. says, "Let's see if you can get all the rings off the stick."

RESPONSE OF CHILD

Affective Reaction
( ) No change in expression
( ) Cries
( ) Tears
( ) Screams
( ) Smiles
( ) Laughs
( ) Frowns
( ) Bland, neutral expression
( ) Fear
( ) Anger

Verbal Reaction
( ) Says "all right" or
    equivalent
( ) Says "No" or equivalent
( ) Converses appropriately
( ) Pronouns appropriate
( ) Inappropriate verbal response
( ) Echolalia
( ) Pronoun reversal
( ) Babbling
( ) Noises
( ) Silent most of time
( ) Sings
( ) Other
    Describe:

Use of Body
( ) Unscrews ball and takes
    rings off
( ) Needs help in unscrewing
    ball but takes rings off
( ) Handles toy but mouths,
    shakes, spins, throws, or
    ————.
( ) Refuses to touch toy
( ) Other
    Describe:

Eye Contact
( ) Above-average eye contact
( ) Average eye contact
( ) Below-average eye contact
( ) No eye contact

Attention to Activity
( ) Concentrated in activity
( ) Attention wanders
( ) Pays no attention to activity

4. E. mixes rings up on floor. E. says, "Show me the smallest ring."

( ) Does as requested ———— Larger ring ———— Smaller
    ring ———— Picks up rings
( ) Doesn't touch
( ) Other
    Describe:

5. E. says, "Show me the biggest ring."
   ( ) Does as requested ——— Larger ring ——— Smaller ring ——— Picks up rings
   ( ) Doesn't touch
   ( ) Other
       Describe:

6. E. says, "Show me a green ring."
   ( ) Does as requested ——— Another color ——— Picks up rings
   ( ) Doesn't touch
   ( ) Other
       Describe:

7. E. says, "Show me a red ring."
   ( ) Does as requested ——— Another color ——— Picks up rings
   ( ) Doesn't touch
   ( ) Other
       Describe:

8. E. says, "Show me a blue ring."
   ( ) Does as requested ——— Another color ——— Picks up rings
   ( ) Doesn't touch
   ( ) Other
       Describe:

9. E. says, "Show me a yellow ring."
   ( ) Does as requested ——— Another color ——— Picks up rings
   ( ) Doesn't touch
   ( ) Other
       Describe:

10. E. says, "Show me a purple ring."
   ( ) Does as requested ——— Another color ——— Picks up rings
   ( ) Doesn't touch
   ( ) Other
      Describe:

11. E. says, "Show me an orange ring."
   ( ) Does as requested ——— Another color ——— Picks up rings
   ( ) Doesn't touch
   ( ) Other
      Describe:

12. E. says, "Put all the rings back on the stick the way they were when I gave it to you."
   ( ) Does as requested
   ( ) Doesn't touch
   ( ) Other
      Describe:

13. To girl: "Let's play with the dolls and doll toys." Play at dolls for 5 minutes. E. joins in play.

REPONSE OF CHILD

Affective Reaction
( ) No change in expression
( ) Cries
( ) Tears
( ) Screams
( ) Smiles
( ) Laughs
( ) Frowns
( ) Bland, neutral expression
( ) Fear
( ) Anger

Verbal Reaction
( ) Says "all right" or equivalent
( ) Says "no" or equivalent
( ) Converses appropriately
( ) Inappropriate verbal response
( ) Echolalia
( ) Pronoun reversal
( ) Babbling
( ) Noises
( ) Sings
( ) Silent most of time
( ) Other
      Describe:

Use of Body

( ) Plays imaginatively and lets E. play
( ) Plays imaginatively but alone
( ) Long chains of different activities with dolls
( ) Short chains of different activities with dolls
( ) Only simple combinations and little or no chaining of activities
( ) Picks up doll or other toy but mouths, shakes, spins, throws, or _____
( ) Does not touch doll or doll toys
( ) Other
     Describe:

Eye Contact

( ) Above-average eye contact
( ) Average eye contact
( ) Below-average eye contact
( ) No eye contact

Attention to Activity

( ) Absorbed in doll play the whole time
( ) Goes to other toys at times but comes back to doll play
( ) Abandons doll play soon
( ) Minutes spent in doll play:

14. To boy: "Let's play cowboy and Indians."

RESPONSE OF CHILD

Affective Reaction

( ) No change in expression
( ) Cries
( ) Tears
( ) Screams
( ) Smiles
( ) Laughs
( ) Frowns
( ) Bland, neutral expression
( ) Fear
( ) Anger

Verbal Reaction

( ) Says "all right" or equivalent
( ) Says "no" or equivalent
( ) Converses appropriately
( ) Inappropriate verbal response
( ) Echolalia
( ) Pronoun reversal
( ) Babbling
( ) Noises
( ) Sings
( ) Silent most of time
( ) Other
     Describe:

Use of Body
( ) Plays imaginatively and lets E. play
( ) Plays imaginatively but alone
( ) Long chains of different activities with props
( ) Short chains of different activities with props
( ) Only simple combinations and little or no chaining of activities
( ) Picks up gun or holster, cowboy hat, bow and arrow, or headdress but mouths, shakes, spins, throws, or ———
( ) Does not touch any of cowboy or Indian toys
( ) Other
    Describe:

Eye Contact
( ) Above-average eye contact
( ) Average eye contact
( ) Below-average eye contact
( ) No eye contact

Attention to Activity
( ) Absorbed in cowboy and/or Indian play the whole time
( ) Goes to other toys at times but comes back to game
( ) Abandons cowboy and/or Indian play soon
( ) Minutes spent in cowboy and/or Indian play:
    ———

Maneuver #5

Examiner gets box of candy placed in clear plastic box, which in turn is placed in another opaque box. Both lids have to be maneuvered to be opened. E. says to child, "There is some candy in this box. You may have one piece." E. puts box on low table. If child continues previous activity, E. takes box to child. If child still ignores, E. opens lid and shows child transparent box.

RESPONSE OF CHILD
Affection Reaction
( ) No change in expression
( ) Cries
( ) Tears
( ) Screams
( ) Smiles
( ) Laughs
( ) Frowns
( ) Bland, neutral expression
( ) Fear
( ) Anger

Verbal Reaction
( ) Starts appropriate conversation
( ) Speaks words, phrases, sentences appropriately
( ) Echolalia
( ) Pronoun reversal
( ) Babbling
( ) Noises
( ) Sings
( ) Silent most of time
( ) Other
    Describe:

Activity with Candy
( ) Ignores candy
( ) Plays with candy
( ) Eats candy:
    ( ) greedily
    ( ) spits part of
       it out
    ( ) eats with enjoy-
       ment, but not
       greedily
    ( ) eats candy wrapper
( ) Dumps candy out
( ) Saves candy (e.g., puts
    in pocket)
( ) Takes paper off
    ( ) puts in wastebasket
( ) Other
    Describe:

Eye Contact
( ) Above-average eye
    contact
( ) Average eye
    contact
( ) Below-average eye
    contact
( ) No eye contact

Opaque Cover
( ) Does not touch
( ) Throws box
( ) Opens
( ) Asks E. to open
( ) Pulls E.'s hand to
    box
( ) Tries to open but
    fails
( ) Other
    Describe:

Transparent Cover
( ) Does not touch after E.
    opens opaque box
( ) Throws box
( ) Takes box out of opaque
    box
( ) Opens
( ) Asks E. to open
( ) Takes E.'s hand and puts
    on box or pulls to box
( ) Tries to open but fails
( ) Other
    Describe:

Maneuver #6

Examiner says to child, "Let's see how big you are." E., while sitting in chair, picks up child and holds child in lap. Talks to child for no more than a minute, then rocks child. Use this time to develop any kind of conversation with child E. wishes to pursue. Child may want to leave E.'s lap and should be allowed to do so. This is a good time to pursue examination of conflict areas in the child.

Response of Child

Affective Reaction

( ) No change in expression
( ) Cries
( ) Tears
( ) Screams
( ) Smiles
( ) Laughs
( ) Frowns
( ) Bland, neutral expression
( ) Fear
( ) Anger

Physical Reaction

( ) Immediately struggles to get away
( ) Sits for little while, then gets off lap
( ) Sits contentedly and allows E. to rock and sing
( ) Sits until E. starts to rock
( ) Sits until E. starts to sing
( ) Other
    Describe:

Verbal Reaction

( ) Starts appropriate conversation at age level
( ) Converses but below age level
( ) Can't answer questions
( ) Can answer questions
( ) Says "yes"
( ) Says "no"
( ) Nods yes
( ) Nods no
( ) Speaks words, phrases, sentences appropriately
( ) Echolalia
( ) Pronoun reversal
( ) Babbling
( ) Noises
( ) Sings
( ) Silent most of time
( ) Other
    Describe:

Eye Contact

( ) Above-average eye contact
( ) Average eye contact
( ) Below-average eye contact
( ) No eye contact

Maneuver #7

Examiner asks child: "Will you sit at the table and draw?" E. places crayons and paper on table and asks child to draw: (1) a straight line, (2) a circle, (3) a cross, (4) parallel lines, (5) a triangle, (6) a square, (7) a diamond, and (8) a person. All will be demonstrated by E. if child fails to draw after being requested to do so. Score 0 if child refuses to draw at all; 1 if scribbles; 2 if draws after demonstration; 3 if draws after verbal request. Score age level of geometric drawings. Score drawing of person by Goodenough system.

RESPONSE OF CHILD

Affective Reaction

( ) No change in expression
( ) Cries
( ) Tears
( ) Screams
( ) Smiles
( ) Laughs
( ) Frowns
( ) Bland, neutral expression
( ) Fear
( ) Anger

Verbal Reaction

( ) Starts appropriate
conversation
( ) Says "yes"
( ) Says "no"
( ) Nods yes
( ) Nods no
( ) Speaks words, phrases,
sentences appropriately
( ) Echolalia
( ) Pronoun reversal
( ) Babbling
( ) Noises
( ) Sings
( ) Silent most of time
( ) Other
Describe:

To Sitting at Table

( ) Will not sit even after E.
physically places child there
( ) Sits at table after E. puts
child there
( ) Sits at table on
verbal request
( ) Sits on E.'s lap

To Drawing Request

( ) Ignores crayons
( ) Throws or drops them on floor
( ) Will not hold crayon when placed
in hand
( ) Picks up crayon spontaneously
( ) Chews crayon
( ) Plays with them
( ) Lines them up
( ) Other
Describe:

Eye Contact

( ) Above-average
eye contact
( ) Average eye contact
( ) Below-average
eye contact
( ) No eye contact

( ) Draws
- ( ) straight lines
- ( ) circle
- ( ) cross
- ( ) parallel lines
- ( ) triangle
- ( ) square
- ( ) diamond
- ( ) person

Maneuver #8

Examiner observes activity or object child likes most during preceding observation. E. reintroduces object or sets stage again for favorite activity. After child is immersed in manipulating object or in activity, E. will take object away from child or prevent child from continuing his activity. E. says, "Show me something in this room you like. . . . Now I'm going to take it away and you try to get it back." Ask: "What do you say?" or "What is the magic word?" if child continues just to reach for object or to cry.

The time after end of structured interview may be used for many purposes, e.g., (1) physical or neurological exam; (2) keeping promise to child to play longer or with something again; (3) repeating certain section of interview.

RESPONSE OF CHILD

Affective Reaction
- ( ) No change in expression
- ( ) Cries
- ( ) Tears
- ( ) Screams
- ( ) Smiles
- ( ) Laughs
- ( ) Frowns
- ( ) Bland, neutral expression
- ( ) Fear
- ( ) Anger

Verbal Reaction
- ( ) Starts appropriate conversation
- ( ) Says "please"
- ( ) Says "thank you"
- ( ) Nods yes
- ( ) Nods no
- ( ) Speaks words, phrases, sentences appropriately
- ( ) Echolalia
- ( ) Pronoun reversal
- ( ) Babbling
- ( ) Noises
- ( ) Sings
- ( ) Silent most of time
- ( ) Other
    Describe:

Physical Reaction

( ) Pulls at or reaches
    for object
( ) Pulls at E.'s arm or
    foot or body
( ) Goes to some other
    toy or inanimate object
( ) Manipulates own body
( ) Sits
( ) Hands toys or other
    objects to E.
( ) Runs or paces around room
( ) Other
    Describe:

Eye Contact

( ) Above-average
    eye contact
( ) Average eye contact
( ) Below-average
    eye contact
( ) No eye contact

If the examiner will review his data from the eight maneuvers, he will find that each of them sheds home light upon the eleven items of the mental status report. Of course, we would expect a limited number of very unsophisticated coping mechanisms. A 2- or 3-year-old will be unable to demonstrate any more than a rudimentary sense of right and wrong and cannot verbalize superego ideals. Such young children cannot openly discuss problems but their play and reactions often imply a surprising awareness of environmental conflicts and tensions. The eight maneuvers reveal much about early object relations and identifications.

In the summary of interviews, either free play or the structured eight maneuvers of DeMyer, one should report: (1) Relationship to E. and parents; (2) Verbal behavior; (3) Use of toys and inanimate objects; (4) Use of body; (5) Affective expression; (6) Physical appearance; (7) Age level of geometric and person drawings and handling of toy objects.

Estimate: (1) Social age; (2) Verbal age; (3) Adaptive age (mean of #7 above); (4) Motor age. (See cases of Billy, p. 81, and Steven, pp. 81-82, for illustrations of the narrative summary for a structured interview with a nonverbal child.)

EARLY DEVELOPMENTAL DEVIATIONS

Before leaving the discussion of preschoolers, it is important to emphasize that these youngsters are in the midst of very rapid developmental processes which have a wide range of variability at any given age level. Too often the mental status even when combined with a careful history fails to answer the questions of parents or the examination itself may raise several additional important issues.

The very young personality is still in such a fluid state that mental and emotional upsets usually do not manifest themselves by the more clear-cut disorders that are common in older children and adults. (See Chapter 9 on nosological diagnoses.) Most often the issue with this age group is not to determine the presence or absence of a specific psychiatric disorder. Rather, the concerns are about his level and rate of development. Biological factors contribute prominently to developmental deviations. In addition, the developmental process in the young organisms is highly susceptible to physical and psychological stresses. Should developmental deviation be present the immediate questions of the clinician as well as the parents are: "Is this a mere lag in developmental rate still within the range of normal variation? Is the deviation an arrest in development or a regression in response to a self-limiting stress? Or is the deviation a more or less permanent one which has ominous implications for the child's future mental and social adjustment?" A conclusion about the child's intellectual level or potential is urgently desired, even demanded. Less often parents want to know if he will become "delinquent" or "neurotic."

Faced with these dilemmas we should call upon our colleagues in clinical psychology. It must be recognized, however, that the psychologist's examination instruments also have serious limitations. DeMyer[20] points out that none of the "currently used standardized psychological test(s) for preschool children can come up with a reliable profile of intellectual, verbal, perceptual-motor, and motor performance over sufficiently wide mental age ranges." Some tests are useful for children under 2½ years of age and others can be used only at the nursery and kindergarten level. DeMyer *et al.*[20] report their own developmental profile which is largely comprised of items from thirteen previously standardized and well-known infant and preschool tests.

It is safe to say that no preschool developmental test can very accurately predict intellectual potential. The so-called I.Q. tests such as the Binet and Wechsler were originally standardized and continue to be used with school-age children for the express purpose of predicting the child's ability to perform in the academic situation. Many mental functions necessary for school performance simply cannot be assessed at the preverbal and early verbal stages. Most investigators and clinicians believe developmental rate and level probably are significantly related in some ways to subsequent I.Q. ratings. However, the exact correlations between specific development parameters and later academic performance factors continue to elude us.

In our society if we erroneously label a child as "mentally retarded" we run a serious risk of "sentencing" the child with a "self-fulfilling prophecy." The various preschool tests can give a better estimate of the child's developmental levels than can nonstandardized clinical observations. Repeated testing at 6-month to yearly intervals can provide our only information about developmental rate. The clinician must help the parents accept that long term study is the only method for answering their questions. After several years of trying to promote healthy development to the best of our ability in a particular child, the ultimate prognosis may become obvious.

With the present state of our knowledge we cannot predict neurosis, delinquency, or social adaptability. However, we can identify early affective, social, and integrative deviations as well as environmental phenomenon known to be frequently present in the early history of socially and psychologically maladapted individuals. When such findings are present in a preschool child, treatment on both an ameliorative and preventive basis is indicated. (See the case of Granville A, p. 148.)

Children who suffer both serious physical and psychological deviations or stresses early in life are most challenging from the diagnostic and prognostic viewpoint. An example of such a case is reviewed below.

CONGENITAL DEFORMITIES AND DEVELOPMENTAL DEVIATIONS

Name: R. T.

Birth Date: 9-21-69   Age: 27 months

Presenting Problem:

Head banging, rejecting, slow development

History:

R. was made a ward of Z. County shortly after birth. History of the natural parents is unavailable. He usually resides in a temporary foster home in his local county 200 miles from the Medical Center. He has a congenital cleft lip and palate. Following each of three surgical corrections he has convalesced in the home of Mrs. N. in this city.

Mrs. N. and the plastic surgeon requested psychiatric consultation because of R.'s slow development in communication, rejecting attitudes toward others, and head banging. Mrs. N. reports the child's personality changed markedly during his last stay in his hometown. He now shows negativism toward her and refuses to eat solid foods. In spite of R's obvious good nutrition, Mrs. N. expressed great concern that the welfare department may take R. and other foster children from her if they do not eat properly. She naively revealed her practice of mixing vitamins and nutriments in milk and giving R. a bottle with a large-hole nipple prior to bringing him to the table for his solid foods. She seemed alarmed at the suggestion the bottles be discontinued. (Mrs. N. has been previously evaluated in this clinic upon referral of another of her foster children. Child Guidance Case #R-9156.)

Mental Status of Child:

R. is a fair boy with multiple bruises. He initially relates very poorly, backing away from the interviewer, and going into rocking behavior, back and forth and side to side on his feet.

By the end of an hour he will interact, sit on the interviewer's lap, show a social smile, sometimes laugh when others in the room do, as well as play ball and use toys with the interviewer. He shows some spontaneous interest in toys. Behavioral observations include:

plays ball for a few throws, rolling ball on floor to interviewer

kisses rag doll

clumsily turns toy telephone dial to produce ringing

will not come when called or when arms offered

sits pliantly on lap or allows self to be held

sometimes responds to name

vocal sounds below 8 or 9 month level, no speech or pseudospeech

interest in toys and objects usually short

much releasing and throwing behavior

maintains rocking behavior for long periods

able to stoop and pick up large ball

infantile grasp

laughs at some play with interviewer — ball

R. is very pliable and compliant to physical manipulation. Spontaneous action is much lower than normal. He showed much resistance to Mrs. N.'s overtures to him during the interview. Interviewer, by being calmer and gentler, was related to somewhat more positively. Foster mother says child relates poorly and screams when being touched by the rest of her family, except 18-month-old grandchild who also is the only person who can get child to laugh.

Psychological Study, 12-14-71:

R. is a 2-year-old boy who was seen to determine his level of intellectual and social functioning.

He is a rather unattractive looking child, his face disfigured by a recent operation; his arms were in splints to prevent his handling the scar. He made no protest at being taken to the interview room and in fact, his only visible acknowledgment of my presence was to allow me to take his hand. This lack of social contact with his environment was very characteristic of his behavior during this meeting. He never smiled nor responded interpersonally with me. When I told him to look me in the eyes, he did not seem to hear. He was willing to sit up in my lap, but showed no affect in this position. When left to himself, R. rocked back and forth on his feet in a repetitive self-stimulating manner.

The following are brief descriptions of R.'s behavior during this meeting: was not able to hold crayon or draw; did not immediately attend to bell that was rung by his left ear; showed no signs of imitation; did not respond to verbal commands; was able to pick up block and find rattle that had been hidden under a box; produced no recognizable language although did make gurgling noises; motor movements generally slow and jerky; enjoyed picking up an object, throwing it, and then retrieving it. These observations of R.'s behavior could be summarized by saying that he is quite retarded in areas of language, motor and social development. It was not possible to obtain an I.Q. score on him because his lack of social contact precluded his following instructions. However, a Vineland Social Maturity Scale was obtained from R.'s foster mother of 6 months. Although there is reason to suspect the accuracy of some of this woman's responses, her information indicated R. has a social maturity age level between 11 months and 1 year. He is thus functioning 1 year below his age level.

Summary of R.'s Evaluation at 2 years, 3 months:

This child is approximately 1 year below his chronological age in intellectual and social development. In addition, he shows signs of emotional tension such as social withdrawal, rocking behavior, excessive crying, negativism, passivity, head banging and refusal to eat solid foods. It is not possible to state at this age how much his delayed development is due to low native intellectual ability and how much is secondary to his emotional state.

His foster mother is extremely well-meaning and interested. However, she is a very tense, anxious person for a variety of reasons, and gives the rather typical picture of the over-protective mother. While it would be unfair, and not substantiated by objective data to say that Mrs. N. is in any way the cause of the delayed development, it is our impression that her tenderheartedness, personal anxiety and over-protectiveness make it seem doubtful that she can give the child the calm environment and the gentle persuasive training he needs to help him become more sociable and learn to do things for himself. The Occupational Therapy Department at this hospital evaluated this child last May and Mrs. N. has not had any success with the techniques they recommended for improving R.'s behavior.

Recommendations:

1. Transfer to a calmer home, hopefully as a permanent placement. This may not be *the* answer for R., but it is certainly worth trying at this point.
2. This child, in our judgment, should be adopted only if the prospective parents are fully aware of his uncertain developmental potential. His chances of reaching a completely average developmental level are questionable. They should also be aware of the genetic risk of cleft palate offspring of this child.
3. His placement in a foster or adoptive home should be with parents who are very patient, do not have high expectations or drive toward training the child, yet can exert gentle, continuous pressure for R. to learn to eat solid foods and perform other self-help and social tasks.
4. Re-evaluate his mental state in 6 months.

Diagnosis: Undetermined—definite slow development.
Psychological Study, 5-8-72, Re-evaluation:

R. has been in a new foster home for the last 2 months. He is much less anxious and withdrawn than he was during the previous evaluation, although he still is not producing any intelligible language. He is currently able to respond interpersonally in that he will make eye contact and will roll a ball back and forth to another person. It was felt that R. is still probably functioning in the retarded range, but testing was not deemed feasible at this time.

It is recommended that R. be re-evaluated in 6 months, at which time it may be possible to more accurately assess the degree of retardation present in this boy. In addition, speech therapy is recommended in the hopes of stimulating language behavior.

Re-evaluation, 11-6-72:

R., now age 3 years, 1½ months, was brought by his foster parents for re-evaluation of his developmental level as requested by our department and for a follow-up appointment in Plastic Surgery. R. has been in this foster home for 6 months and it is considered a permanent placement.

Observations of the Child:

Comparing R. with previous examinations last May and 11 months ago, he has made a number of gains, particularly in the area of sociability. He was noted to still rock from one side to the other while standing on his feet, but this was minimal as compared with 1 year ago. He separated from his foster mother without a reaction. However, she soon came after him, saying she thought he should be taken to the bathroom first and on the second separation he cried and was obviously angry at being separated from her.

In the playroom he at first rejected all toys. He made a whining "Ma" or "Mama" sound as he went to and looked searchingly at the playroom door. However, he soon settled down and I was able to get a good bit of eye contact and non-verbal communication from him. I was unable to get any intelligible speech other than the "Mama" but he would take my hand or make gestures for the things he wanted. For example, he couldn't figure how to get the doors open on a big truck after I had shown him three times. He would close the doors and then come and get my hand for me to open them again for him. When I insisted he could open the doors himself he did so and seemed extremely pleased. He then played for awhile repeating the opening and closing of the doors to the truck. He would be easily frustrated if they did not open immediately and cried briefly. Episodically he would stop his play and go to the door, apparently searching for his mother. He understood simple directions and obeyed me.

After briefly rolling some trucks around the floor he climbed into the sand box and played there as a 1- to 1½-year-old child would do. He would pat and hit the sand, run it through his fingers and would pick it up with the sand on the back of his hands. He briefly paid attention to the toys in the sand box but most of the time was spent running his hands through the sand. He then began to throw sand, but stopped when I asked him to. He then engaged in some teasing behavior in which he would pick up some sand and gesture as if to throw it, look at me and then giggle when I told him not to. He still mouths toys and he tried to eat the sand. In general he was much more friendly and sociable with me. He rejected my attempts to get him to use crayon or pencil.

Interview with the Parents, 11-6-72:

The parents were seen together with their social worker. These parents have a great deal of positive involvement with R. and are extremely pleased with his development. They would like to believe that the improvement of the last 6 or 8 months means that he is intellectually normal. The mother reported that he is now feeding himself, able to drink from a glass, engages in emotional interaction with the family as well as with other children, can say Mama, Dad and Hi and is toilet trained. He is attending a nursery school 2½ hours per day 5 days per week and also receiving speech therapy at this school (a school report has been requested). The foster parents intend to adopt this child when he has completed his surgery.

Summary and Recommendations for 11-6-72:

R. has made considerable progress, particularly in the social and human interaction area but has not made much progress in his speech development. His play behavior and play interests still appear to be that of a child between 18 months and 2 years of age. He is toilet trained and is able to understand and usually follows directions. He appears to this examiner to be a much more relaxed and comfortable child than he was a year ago.

The foster parents were told that we strongly suspect this child is mentally retarded but that it may be mild. At this point we cannot give them an actual I.Q. level nor any prediction regarding the upper limits of his developmental potential. R. will be hospitalized for surgery in January. We have requested that he be admitted to the hospital 1 day early for a prolonged period of observation and another attempt to do standardized developmental tests on him.

Psychological Study, 1-19-73:

Attempted Cattell Infant Intelligence Scale, 1-10-73
Developmental Profile, 1-12-73

Referral:

R. was seen for a re-assessment of his social and intellectual development. Initial evaluations indicated that R. was approximately 1 year below his chronological age (3 years, 4 months) in intellectual and social development. Additionally, signs of emotional tensions were noted in this child as he engaged in excessive crying, rocking behavior, passivity, withdrawal and head banging. Later evaluations reported a steady decrease in emotional behaviors along with an increase in the level of social responsivity. The present study was initiated as an attempt to further clarify this child's intellectual development.

Behavior Notes, 1-19-73:

R. separated from his parents to go to the examining room with no protest. He did indicate, by his initial coolness toward the examiner and by short glances back toward his parents, that he would have preferred to stay on the ward with them. At times during the examining hour he actually would go to the door, sometimes pulling the examiner with him, and say "Mama." These behaviors are of note because of the extreme passivity this youngster exhibited in the past.

R. spent most of the hour moving about the room, going in and out of the door or walking up and down the hall. It was impossible to engage his interest in a task, a toy, or other activity for more than just a few seconds. He would respond to verbal directions but there was no sustained effort in his responses. No rocking or similar activity was noted during the hour. R. indicated his awareness of the examiner throughout the period. For instance, he would never wander very far away and would return quickly if the examiner was out of his sight.

Test Results, 1-19-73:

Items of the Cattell Scale were administered. The results were so variable, however, that no scoring was attempted. On many of the items that he did not pass, it was impossible to tell if he was unable to do the task or simply would not put out sufficient effort to complete it. Some of the activities that he did engage in were as follows:
1. responded to and followed out some simple commands
2. picked up cubes and placed them in a cup
3. built a tower out of three or more blocks
4. scribbled spontaneously with a pencil

Generally, R. did not succeed on any of the items above the 2 year level, but *seemed* capable of completing many tasks below that level. The Developmental Profile Assessment, based on maternal report, places R.'s general developmental level at about 14 months below his chronological age. The social level was his relatively highest area, but, it should be noted, this doesn't reflect the "emotional" quality that is yet a part of his social behavior (*i.e.*, short attention, etc.). R's communicative (most particularly verbal) skills were not only much below age level but were also significantly below R.'s own general level of development.

Conclusions:

R.T.'s mental status appears to be showing continued improvement since he was initially evaluated. Social responsive behaviors are apparently on the increase while many emotional behaviors (*i.e.*, rocking, head banging, etc.) are decreasing. Additionally, he has achieved many self-help skills such as self-feeding, undressing, etc., and can indicate his desire to use the toilet and does so with but few accidents. He does make some response to simple verbal directions.

The present data indicate that R. is still approximately 1 year behind in general and intellectual development. Any predictions about his later intellectual abilities must yet be considered as very tentative due to present emotional factors such as short attention and lack of sustained effort that make clear assessment of his abilities impossible, and because of the general unreliability of measures taken at this level of development as predictors of later performance. The best *guess* of this examiner at this time is that R. will be able to go to school (particularly if a strong program of speech therapy is carried out over the next 2 or 3 years) but will probably require special education classes. Again, this is a tentative prediction based on inconclusive evidence.

Recommendations:

1. It seems apparent that R.'s foster parents are providing very much the kind of day-to-day home environment that R. needs. That is, they seem to combine the warmth and personal respect R. deserves with the gentle firmness that he needs. Without this firmness, R. is likely not to engage in many of the activities which he is capable of and should be engaging in. His foster parents should continue to demand *gradual* increments in responsive behavior. For instance, he wouldn't be expected right away to put on his coat and button it, but he might be able to help by extending his arms or even slipping his arms into the sleeves as a first step.

2. R.'s verbal behavior is the outstanding area in which extensive professional help is needed. His communicative level is significantly below his general level of development. One-to-one contact with a professional speech therapist on an almost daily basis seems badly needed to stimulate and shape verbal behaviors. Short attention span could also be dealt with in that context. R.'s foster parents seem very open to professional direction and could greatly assist a speech therapy program by employing speech-eliciting techniques at home under the direction of R.'s speech therapist. It is recommended that a fairly intensive long-term speech therapy program be immediately considered or that his present program at the Rehabilitation Center be augmented if possible.

At the time of R.'s last evaluation, his improved social development indicated that the emotional disorder which was impairing his development had been at least partially relieved. His very poor language development remained and his rate of overall progress was obviously retarded. This slow rate points to the likelihood that his schooling cannot be accomplished in regular classes and he will need special education procedures. However, we still do not know his ultimate potential and the decision about classroom placement can and should be deferred for another 2 or 3 years. It is important that R. now has permanent parents in a stable home. These parents have been included in R.'s evaluation each step of the way. They are fully aware of the child's developmental problems. While they maintain a good degree of optimism, they appear to be free of unrealistic expectations which could produce future serious family stress.

To some readers, R.'s case may seem extreme and unusual. However, children with similar clinical pictures are referred for psychiatric evaluation with considerable frequency. Often these children have been previously diagnosed as suffering Infantile Autism, severe Mental Retardation, or both. The evidence of serial examinations of R. indicates that either diagnosis is probably erroneous. These particular diagnostic labels can instill an attitude of profound pessimism. Therefore, a definitive diagnostic label must be deferred unless the clinical findings are so obvious and conclusive that the clinician is left no alternative. The goals in cases such as R.T. are to help the guardians sustain an attitude of conservative optimism, meet problems only as they arise, and institute remedial procedures only when the child appears ready to benefit from them. Parents usually need help in treading the narrow line between over-protective infantilization and excessive pressure for achievement, both of which can impede the child's developmental progress.

SUMMARY

The examination of preschool children, especially if they have limited speech development, is quite difficult. These children must be examined within a developmental frame of reference rather than from the standpoint of differentiating specific mental disorders. The examiner must try to estimate the child's social age, verbal age, adaptive age and motor age. The eight maneuvers of DeMyer are presented as a structured procedure for examining this age group. Data from this examination can be related to the mental status outline with special attention to the developmental levels.

Mental disturbances in preschool children are most clearly manifested by deviations in development and parents are usually worried about the possibility of mental retardation and future inability to learn in school. Both emotional stress and biological factors can interfere with early development. The differentiation of these two alternative causations can be extremely difficult. In fact, many times biological and social factors are simultaneously interacting to produce the clinical manifestations of developmental impairment. Pinpointing the exact etiology and prognosticating can be virtually impossible. The child's developmental level and rate must be studied by serial examinations. The clinician must assist the parents in correcting any pathogen which is rectifiable and in presenting properly timed remedial measures. A case with serious developmental deviations as a result of biological deformities and emotional deprivation is presented to illustrate these points.

Chapter 5

MENTAL STATUS PROFILES, NORMAL AND ABNORMAL

THE EMPHASIS of this text has been upon the diagnostic assessment of children rather than on a review of the established and theoretical knowledge about various nosological categories. The reader should keep in mind that appraisal of the ego functions of a specific child is useful only in estimating the severity of his illness. Such appraisals cannot be used as a basis for diagnostic classification, since classification includes etiological and prognostic considerations which are not evident from the mental status examination alone.

Unfortunately, it is easier to measure degrees of dysfunction than relative states of health. It would be impossible and presumptuous to attempt to draw a "normal" mental status profile for every age level. However, a discussion of the extremes of distortion seen in clinical practice and the range of normal variability for the ego functions listed in the preceding chapter seems feasible. Some generalizations about age-appropriateness of behavior, the significance of quantitative aberrations, and various combinations of ego deficits are also possible.

THREE PRESCHOOL BOYS

The following three preschool youngsters behaved quite differently on examination. The fact that each of them was referred because of "suspected infantile autism" is illustrative of the confusion which has arisen over the term "autism," even in sophisticated circles. The reader is asked to compare these children not only in terms of their total behavior but in terms of which ego functions were impaired and the extent of their impairment.

Mental Status Examinations

PETE, AGE 2½ YEARS. Pete was met in the waiting room. He smiled and went eagerly to the playroom, taking my hand. He talked spontaneously in complete sentences and could be well understood. He expressed an interest in the water and then went about the room examining the toys, settling for a baby doll. He asked me to put a bib on the doll and fix a bottle for her. He then fed her. After a period of this he went to the doll house, took out the furniture, and placed it on a play table. He identified the various pieces of furniture and commented about some of the broken ones being unusable. He complained of the icebox being broken, too, but accepted the explanation that it was just a toy, not designed to be opened. After some ten minutes of doll play, he went to the sandbox and took a car out of it. He then reached and complained that he couldn't get a plane out. This was obtained for him, and he complained that he couldn't get another plane. He was asked if he wanted to get in the sandbox, and he said he did. Permission was given and he climbed into the sandbox, climbing in and out many times, playing enthusiastically with the planes and with the sand. He would make the planes fly and land with appropriate noises and sometimes would stop and spontaneously identify the various parts of the plane. After a period of sand play he went about the room, enthusiastically examining the many other toys he found. He asked for some clay and played with it for a while, explaining, "You don't eat this." He then returned to the baby and bottle, playing with them for a while.

I asked Pete to draw for me, and he was very resistive to this, wanting to go back to his own play. However, he did cooperate after a few minutes and was able to copy a line and a circle, but he complained that he couldn't copy a box and he refused to try to draw a figure.

He was observed in some spontaneous play with his sister for a few minutes. They played quite easily together for a short time and then began to fight over the toys. It was noticed that Pete held his own and the sister began to cry. The mother came up and complained that they were embarrassing her. She separated them and said that she would take care of them when she got home.

BILLY, AGE 2 YEARS, 5 MONTHS. Billy is an attractive child, appearing sturdy and well built and with good muscular coordination. Alone with me in the examination room he was extremely upset at being separated from his mother. Because I could not console him, I asked the mother to join me in the examination. He sat on her lap, or extremely close to her feet when he was on the floor. As soon as he was comfortable and sure that I was not going to separate him from his mother again, he became interested in the toys. He played with a total of seven different toys, using all of them appropriately. He pushed the lawn mower back and forth on the floor. He played the musical book briefly. He asked his mother to read from the animal noise book and pulled the strings to make the animal sounds after his mother showed him how to do it. He took the top off the Tinker Toys and put a stick in a wheel. He tried to spin a top, unsuccessfully, because the top was broken. He pushed the train briefly and played with the wind-up bear three different times. He perceived the winding mechanism, tried to wind it unsuccessfully, then handed the toy to me to get it working.

In the drawing maneuver he sat on his mother's lap, picked up a crayon spontaneously, drew a straight line after demonstration, and scribbled after I demonstrated a circle. He used a circular motion after I demonstrated it but was never able to draw just individual circles.

I frustrated Billy by taking candy away from him. He was able to use a socially appropriate method of getting the candy from me by asking me please to give him the candy.

STEVEN, AGE 3 YEARS, 4 MONTHS. Steven is a chunky, willful child of enormous strength who can go quickly from one emotion to another. He could fly into an angry withdrawal, only to smile happily the next moment. With his mother, he was the same. When he kicked at her, she told him to stop and held his legs firmly. Then she smiled and tickled him, and he responded with a giggle. Once he retreated under the couch during the neurological examination, and she lured him out merely by rolling the toy sweeper beside him. If he wanted something, he could generally be distracted by some other object.

His approach to me was sometimes babyish and sometimes

4

bizarre. On first coming to my office, he reacted with fear to the movie camera and took refuge behind my chair. When I turned my head toward him and said something reassuring, he put his fingers on my eyelids, an action he often does at home with his parents and his dog.

Steven's response to adaptive tasks was as follows:

a. Ball play — he refused, although he picked up the ball after a pointing cue.

b. Ring stack set — he took rings off stick but gave no indication that he understood the names of sizes or colors; his repositioning the rings was done well with some attention to size, and he made several corrections showing some appreciation of the nature of the apparatus. His final position of the rings was not correct.

c. Cowboy and Indian — of the materials offered he accepted with alacrity the horses and cows, lining them in a row. He seemed generally oblivious to my attempts to play but let me parallel play and looked at me.

d. Candy — he opened the opaque box immediately but needed to have the top pulled off the transparent one. He at first played with the M & M's, then ate them after I put one in his mouth. He ignored the wrapped candy. His coordination was adequate.

e. Drawing — he drew a straight line after demonstration. To other requests he made a controlled scribble. He held his crayon in his fist.

His verbal behavior consisted of imitating a train and babbling. He made little effort to communicate with me, although he was not a difficult child to "read." Mostly he wanted to do what he wanted when he wanted, but he could be led with some resistance to try a new task if too much was not demanded. He understood some of what I said. I asked him where his mama was. An anxious expression came to his face. He got off my lap, took my hand, and led me to the door. He seemed to use my physical presence for comfort when he sought it but did not allow me much latitude in my approach to him, preferring to structure the interaction in a strict way.*

---

*The author is indebted to Dr. Marian K. DeMyer for the case material of Billy and Steven.

Comparison of the Mental Status of These Three Boys

The reader who has had no experience observing preschool children in a nonclinical setting is urged to arrange some observation periods as a part of his training. Only through actually watching children of this age group can one develop an appreciation for the wide range of normal behavior and at the same time sense the extremes which are beyond the range of normality. Those experienced with preschoolers will immediately be aware that the mental status examination of Pete, the first child, failed to reveal any striking abnormalities. Steven, the third patient, showed marked abnormal behavior in most areas, and Billy's over-all functioning fell somewhere between that of Pete and Steven. The referral complaints for these boys mentioned periods of severe withdrawal interspersed with episodic emotional outbursts, various misbehaviors, and sleep pattern disruptions. The possibility of "infantile autism" was included in the differential considerations of each of the referring persons. A comparison of the ego functions, as outlined on page 35 of each of these children explicitly differentiates them from one another.

APPEARANCE. The boys do not differ in that each had good physical development and were free of any stigmata or mannerisms.

MOOD OR AFFECT. In this area the differences are quite striking. None of the boys showed obvious sadness, which is an affective expression difficult to differentiate from frustration and anger in a very small child. They all revealed a full range of emotion, from happiness to fear to rage. For Pete the prevailing mood appears to have been contentment in happy—at times exuberant—play, while a tense fearfulness pervaded Billy's interview. Considering his age and the circumstances, Billy's fear would not be considered so unusual. However, this paniclike clinging to the mother persisted during the next five interviews. Steven's moods were so variable and wide-range that one is at a loss to assign a "prevailing" mood to the interview hour. Pete illustrated a smooth, modulated transition from one affect to another, with the changes being readily comprehensible in terms of the immediate environment. By contrast the other boys' emotional expressions were sudden, unpredictable, and more intense. Billy's emotionality was easily modulated by the presence of the mother, while Steven's emotional outbursts were extremely difficult to change.

COPING MECHANISMS.   The boys' methods of handling their feelings, anxieties, and frustrations were immature and numerically few because all of them actually are chronologically immature. In addition to direct expression of angry impulses, all three used or attempted to use evasion, avoidance, and withdrawal to the point of appearing obstinate. However, Billy did this much less when his mother was present, and Pete defied the examiner only once, when the request for figure drawings was beyond his abilities. All of the patients tried to manipulate the environment, but again Pete was by far the most sophisticated. He made direct verbal requests for the examiner's participation and once by strong hints obtained permission to climb into the sandbox. Pete demonstrated awareness of adult restrictions and controlled an impulse to eat clay by offering an adult quotation, "You don't eat this." Neither of the other boys demonstrated this much ability to use the adult for either personal gratification or control of unacceptable wishes.

PERCEPTION AND ORIENTATION.   Each of the boys appeared to be oriented correctly to his own name and to his mother. We do not expect precise orientation to time and place at this age, and these items were not checked. Perceptual ability is also limited at this age; at least, the child's limited language makes it impossible for him to tell us his understanding of the objects and events in his environment. By inference from the children's play it appeared that Steven had the least ability to differentiate the toys by size, color, or appropriate use. It is impossible to tell whether this apparent perceptual deficit was due to poor comprehension, inattention, or lack of motivation to perform.

THOUGHT PROCESSES AND VERBALIZATIONS. Without fairly extensive conversation, it is impossible to ascertain the thinking of another human being. However, when a child is engaged in some activity we can reasonably assume his thought processes are active. Steven's behavior was so unusual and unpredictable that it seems very likely that his thinking was quite unconventional. His verbal ability was similar to that seen in children 8 to 12 months of age. Billy had language ability, but fear and poor motivation reduced his productivity so that the actual vocabulary level remained uncertain.

FANTASY. For preschool children, fantasy play with a paucity of verbal accompaniment is usual. Therefore, attempts to describe these children's fantasies separately from coping or thinking behavior would be redundant. Fantasy content can only be accurately obtained from what the child will or can tell you about his play and dreams.

SUPEREGO. Internalization of the superego is still developing in the 2- to 4-year-old. As was mentioned, only Pete gave clear evidence of being aware of adult "do's and don'ts."

CONCEPT OF SELF AND OBJECT RELATIONS. These boys clearly illustrated different ways of relating to the examiner and to their mother. Relations with peers and other adults were not observed and can only be surmised. All of them made eye contact and permitted touching. Steven's act of putting his finger on the eyelids of the examiner, his parents, and his dog is behavior which is seen infrequently and usually disappears well before 12 months of age. Steven showed relatively little differentiation between his mother and the examiner in his behavior reactions until the examiner specifically mentioned the mother. Billy sharply differentiated between the mother and the examiner and clung to his mother in fear. Such behavior is found commonly at 8 to 10 months, but persistence with such intensity (five interviews) to age 2½ is quite inappropriate. By contrast, the examiner remarked about

Pete, "It was fun to be with him." Psychosexual identifications are hardly measurable at such a young age. It should be noted, however, that Pete's doll-baby play is not unusual for a 2½-year-old boy and cannot be used as a positive or negative sign regarding his psychosexual identity.

Relation of Mental Status to the Final Diagnostic Formulation

The three preschool patients just described received complete diagnostic work-ups, and the final formulations were in accord with the impressions gained from the mental status examinations. From personal and family histories and from additional direct examinations, no positive findings of an organic nature were found in any of the cases.

At the initial interview, Pete's mother denied any significant family problems and gave a very bland, conventional family history. However, in a subsequent interview she was told that Pete seemed to be, psychologically, a rather healthy preschooler. We believed he had the symptoms described by her, and they could only be understood as a reaction to some environmental stress. The mother then told of her own distress about a current extramarital affair of the father's. She had withheld this information out of embarrassment, believing — perhaps hoping — that Pete's lack of direct knowledge of the marital problem would leave him unaffected by it.

Billy's developmental lag was directly related to his pathological attachment and dependence upon the mother. The child's dependence and the mother's overprotectiveness appeared to be the result of a chronically high anxiety level in both of them. There were a variety of severe emotional problems in the family. The child's father and brother both suffered from psychosis, the parents were divorced, and the mother's relationship with her own mother was very tumultuous. While Billy's situation appeared to be a stress reaction causing only moderate impairment, the severity and chronicity of the stress, his tender age, and the poor outlook for future improvement in family relations all pointed toward a relatively poor prognosis.

Those who examined Steven, the third child, agreed on a diagnosis of early childhood schizophrenia with both autistic (Kanner) and symbiotic (Mahler) features. The dynamics for such illnesses are currently under much scientific scrutiny, and the theoretical issues will not be repeated here. An excellent review and explanation of the semantic confusion surrounding childhood schizophrenia is contained in a paper by Hirschberg and Bryant.[37] These authors reviewed and summarized the literature of several leading investigators. Many of the apparent theoretical differences about childhood psychoses are owing to the lack of consensual agreement on definition of terms and to the fact that various researchers have obtained their clinical cases from vastly different sociocultural populations. Childhood schizophrenia is not a disease entity but a syndrome, within which children suffering profound but varied symptoms of diverse etiology are grouped. On playroom examination, Steven exhibited many of the classical signs and symptoms of early childhood psychosis.

TWO SCHOOL-AGE GIRLS

The school initiated the referrals of the two 8-year-old girls whose mental status examinations are reported below. Neither child was making satisfactory academic progress in spite of high average (Abby) and superior intelligence (Jane). The school complained that Abby was so boisterous and destructive in the classroom that she could no longer be contained there. Jane's behavior was exemplary, but she did not seem "to grasp the academic material or know the answers." The school had recommended repeating the third grade for Jane and had requested that Abby be withdrawn from school after her failure to improve in a special class for emotionally disturbed children,

Mental Status Examinations

JANE, AGE 8 YEARS, 5 MONTHS. Jane had no physical abnormalities. She was appropriately dressed and groomed for an 8-year-old. During the family intake conference, Jane sat quietly and did not attempt to speak even when spoken to. She hesitated briefly when asked to come for an individual interview. She entered the play therapy room and stood rooted by the door. She did not turn her head to explore the room visually but only looked at me, occasionally giving a furtive side glance about the room. She refused to sit or explore the room even when invited. She did not speak but only grimaced painfully and wrung her hands fretfully. She would not participate in any games with me and would not move from her fixed position. When I left the room she explored it quickly, painting a female figure and then drawing an excellent reproduction of a horse on the blackboard. She then returned to her original spot and stood there until I re-entered the room. I then attempted to interest her in the doll house, but she refused to talk or move. When I again left the room she rearranged the doll house and resumed her former position before I returned. She eagerly joined her parents at the session's close.

At the second interview one week later, Jane again appeared quite anxious. However, she sat down when invited and talked much more freely. She still wrung her hands and grimaced during the conversation. She enunciated well, but there were occasional gaps in her knowledge. For instance, she did not know when her birthday was but only that it was during school and before the rest of the family's. In comparing Indianapolis and her home town she could only say there were more hospitals and taller buildings in Indianapolis. Jane stated she reads during gym class because she doesn't like to play. She made good grades but her teacher thought she needed help with reading and sounding. She mentioned two bad boys in her room. When asked why they were bad she replied that one makes low marks and the other talks, so they get whipped. She then denied ever being whipped. She related several fears consisting of the following: she's afraid to sleep alone because the trees make shadows on the walls, and she's afraid people look in her upstairs window although she's never seen anyone. She doesn't like to go to the basement to get potatoes because she can't reach the light and some rotten potatoes are slimy. She's afraid to look down when she crosses bridges. She doesn't know how to swim if she should fall in.

Her favorite TV programs are horse stories, war stories, circus acts (her favorite), and the Flintstones. Her best friends are John and Karen, and they play house together frequently. She likes to be the mommy because she bosses and spanks the baby. She does not like to be the baby and will leave the game when she is the baby. She stated she usually dreams of horses and dreams that "Fury" will protect her. She said she always dreams about animals but no humans. She would not elaborate on this. She desires to be a "big kid" so she can get out of school and go to college. She also wants to grow older because when she is 20 she can do anything and her mother can't tell her what to do, but she says it's up to her mother if she gets married or not. She also related when she is 16 she may go on dates — but she doesn't want to go on dates because she is afraid she'll get lost. She then related how scared she was when she once got lost in a grocery store. She looked out the window toward the end of the interview and stated she might climb out on the roof but she was afraid she might get blown away.

Toward the end of the second hour she talked easily and without many overt signs of anxiety. However, she indicated she wanted to terminate the session by asking several times if she couldn't now go out with her mother. She accepted a roll of lemon candy; she did not care to eat any there but wished to take the whole roll home. She sat quietly in the hall until her mother returned.

ABBY, AGE 8½ YEARS. Abby is a dark-haired, rather pale girl of average size with slightly protruding teeth. She has a pseudo-mature manner, pedantically enunciating words with a rather grown-up vocabulary. She gives the appearance of the prissy "good little girl." Conversation was logical and clear but had the quality of repeating just what her mother had said. There were no reversals of pronouns. She was correctly oriented to time, place, and person. She knew she was being brought for examination because of "nervousness." She could not describe how her "nervousness" showed itself or what discomfort, if any, it caused her.

Eye contact was frequent but the relationship was distant. She moved around the room most of the time, talking rapidly in response to questions. When she would stop or sit down to talk with the examiner, there was much fidgeting of hands. High-pitched, inappropriate giggling continued throughout the hour. She was very attentive to the examiner and stayed with assigned tasks such as drawings. When asked about school,

Abby said, "School is dirty. The boys call me retarded. They put me upon a table and pulled my dress up and took pictures. Boys are dirty. The boys next door [they are 3 and 4 years old] come over just when I am napping and make noise." She has no friends. "Mother says boys are rough and boyish." There was a very lonely quality when she said, "Some girls have long hair." This statement was abruptly interjected into the conversation and seemed irrelevant to the question about friendships.

When asked about her relationship with her brother, she responded, "My brother carries me sometimes. I like to be carried all over. I'd like to be a cuddly cat; you would not be lonely and people pet you. I am the baby in the family and I'll always be the baby." Asked what she'd do when grown up, she replied, "I'll be a secretary like you [pause], oh, I'll be a doctor." There was no elaboration of this.

She denied ever getting angry except when she is "nervous." "Then I holler at the devil — dumb old idiot — then I call Mother stupid and other names. She doesn't like it" (much tense high-pitched giggling). She was evasive and vague when asked about her father, saying only that he is "nice" and they have "fun." She couldn't remember any of the activities with which they have "fun." She denied that either she or her father ever got angry and called each other names.

Abby said she spends much time daydreaming "but only of the songs Mother taught me." She talked readily and in great detail about her dreams and fantasies. Indeed, most of the spontaneous conversation consisted of telling dreams or fantasy stories. She did not clearly differentiate her stories from her dreams, making it difficult to know what she was trying to tell the examiner or to know the relevance of her conversation to the activity of the moment or her life situation. Nightmares are very real and come often and, although scary, appear to be enjoyed. "Monsters, creatures, and beings look at me, show me their teeth, and want to eat me. They chase me into the dark forest all the time very close together. They get closer and closer and it is dark as night." She then put the playroom light out with great glee. A Hansel and Gretel theme with a wicked witch was repeated often. These dreams were usually fascinating, with tall trees making everything dark. Her affect while telling these stories is best described as apprehensive yet pleasurable.

Drawings were age-appropriate and were pictures of a family and a witch's house surrounded by big trees. Wishes included (1) to be a bird "so that I'd fly in the air when people chase me," (2) to have some swimming pools "so that I won't have to go to school," and (3) to go to Florida and "swim in the deep deep ocean where it will be dark." She was unable to explain the connection between having swimming pools and not going to school.

Comparison of the Mental Status of These Two Girls

Neither a nosological classification nor a diagnostic formulation is possible on the basis of these mental status interviews alone. However, it should be apparent that both quantitatively and qualitatively Abby demonstrates a greater degree of personality disturbance in the interview situation than Jane does.

APPEARANCE. Neither of the girls showed any outstanding abnormality or difference from each other in their general appearance.

MOOD OR AFFECT. Each of the girls was described by the examiner as appearing fearful and anxious. Both girls demonstrated excessive hand movement. Jane appeared more composed, yet more tense and inhibited. By contrast Abby seemed flighty. Abby demonstrated inappropriate affect as she discussed some of her problems and was unable to verbalize appropriate concern about her feelings. Jane made it clear that her fears were distressful to her. Although apparently too fearful (or possibly too obstinate) to move, she demonstrated both an ability and a partial desire to comply when she quickly and furtively obeyed the examiner's requests while he was out of the room.

ORIENTATION AND PERCEPTION. There was no disturbance reported in orientation to time, place, or person for either of the girls. At no point was there any question about Jane's ability to perceive reality. While Abby does not show a profound disturbance in this area and, if pressed, might well have admitted that such things as boys taking pictures of her genitals had not really happened, she presented these fantasies as if they were a factual answer to the examiner's question about her school adjustment. Again, when asked about her relationship with her brother, she became lost in her own desires to be petted and cuddled, leaving the listener with only the foggiest notion of her brother or what their relationship might be like. She was so absorbed in her fantasies that she showed no concern about the listener's comprehension.

COPING MECHANISMS. During Jane's first hour when she stood rooted to the door, it was not possible to tell if she was frightened or angry about the examination. Her body posture, the fact that she was willing to fulfill the examiner's requests while he was out of the room, and her subsequent telling of her many fears supports the idea that she was quite frightened. She was also frightened of displeasing the teacher, of high places, of being alone, of the dark, and of growing up. At first she handled her fear by constriction and avoidance but by the second hour had overcome much of her fear of the examiner. She appeared to be trying to handle her other fears by intellectualizing in the form of reasoning logically and planning for various eventualities. None of these defense mechanisms can be considered particularly pathological per se. However, her constriction and avoidance may well be responsible for some of her poor performance in school. She is obviously anxious, and therefore her coping mechanisms are not completely successful. Her desires to grow up and emancipate herself from her mother, while at the same time believing her mother will handle major decisions (such as marriage), are not particularly inappropriate for an 8-year-old girl. However, if such notions persist into puberty and adolescence, we would be forced to say that her ability to comprehend adult independent functioning is impaired. Troublesome sexual and aggressive impulses are not discussed directly by Jane, but their presence is implied in her doll play and her concerns about growing up.

In contrast, Abby recounted fears and preoccupation with sexual and aggressive impulses. These impulses were not acted out directly during the examination. She may verbally assault her mother at times, or this could be fantasy. The fact that appropriate affect does not accompany her thoughts is considered by many clinicians to be an unconscious coping device, serving to make such thoughts psychologically tolerable. The unusual amount of fantasy in which the aggressive and sexual themes were reviewed may be considered also a coping mechanism to lessen conscious anxiety. The sexual and aggressive content of her fantasies are only thinly disguised, if at all. Unconscious phenomenon cannot be observed directly but can only be inferred. One cannot be certain that the fantasy and separation of appropriate affect are attempts to cope with anything. Yet, if we accept the premise that sexual and aggressive impulses are common and highly charged human attributes, we must say Abby is quite unusual in her expression of these feelings.

THOUGHT PROCESSES AND VERBALIZATIONS. At first Jane showed a paucity of conversation, but gradually this reached a normal level. As she improved in her ability to converse with the examiner, she demonstrated coherence, logic, and orderliness in her thinking. By contrast, Abby talked readily and in considerably volume from the very beginning. She always responded to the examiner's questions but was quickly stimulated by her own inner thoughts and would elaborate unnecessarily and irrelevantly to inquiries. The examiner did report much of her conversation to be logical and clear, but at those times she seemed to be repeating things her mother had said. Her ability to parrot adults, her appropriate drawings, and her relating of the Hansel and Gretel story indicate that Abby is capable of some conventional thinking.

FANTASY. As was indicated, Abby's fantasies are not in themselves terribly uncommon in childhood. However, they preoccupy her with such intensity that it was hard to get her to attend to other topics. The excessive number of fantasies, coupled with her preoccupation with primitive sexual and aggressive urges, are unusual in an 8-year-old girl. Indeed, if they are not unusual, the ease with which she shares them and the apparent unawareness that such fantasy is not expected from little girls this age are pathological. Abby did not elaborate on her three wishes, so it is difficult to understand their meaning to her. However, the unlikelihood of her wishes being ever fulfilled again points to Abby's tenuous hold on reality.

Jane did not reveal any spontaneous fantasies, and she did not play during the interview situation. However, she did tell about her play with friends in the community. Playing house is certainly a very conventional activity for an 8-year-old girl. In her particular case, the play she described seemed to be on the theme of freeing herself from adult domination by assuming the adult role, bossing and spanking the baby, and refusing to assume the role of the baby in relation to her playmates. She did not elaborate on her dreams, and this examiner does not know the significance of dreams which contain no human beings. However, the fact that Fury, a well-known horse, protects her in her dreams indicate that the dreams must have frightening content. Other wishes she gave in the course of conversation were her desire to grow up, go to college, and be free of her mother's domination. While she fantasies about the prospect of growing up, she also indicated her feelings that there are fears connected with growing up and being free from parents. On the basis of this interview it can be said that Jane is capable of indulging in fantasy, does not do so to excess, perhaps is somewhat constricted in this area, and did not reveal any pathological fantasies.

SUPEREGO. In examining the child and observing his playroom behavior, it is usually much easier to discern defects in his conscience than it is to be certain he has a well internalized concept of right and wrong. Certainly both of these girls manifested an awareness of what society accepts as proper and improper behavior. Even Abby, who had been reported to strike out and be disruptive in school, did not indulge in any overt aggressive behavior in the playroom situation and seemed quite aware of what the adult world considers good and bad behavior. The aggressive and sexual impulses were permitted expression only in fantasy and were rationalized or presented as something beyond her control and not willfully indulged.

CONCEPT OF SELF AND OBJECT RELATIONS. Both girls appeared to appraise the role of the examiner realistically and see him as a helping individual. Jane was initially quite frightened and perhaps negativistic with the examiner, but this is not considered unusual unless it persists over many interviews. Allowance must be made for the newness of the situation. Although the examiner felt Abby was "distant" and could not always be understood, the child gave many signs of trying to establish rapport. On the basis of these observations, one would feel that neither child is completely incapable of making meaningful human relations and each has a desire for closeness with adults. Their relationships are further differentiated, however, when we look at their direct and indirect references to other people in their lives. Jane spontaneously mentioned friends with whom she apparently plays appropriately. She seems to be identified with the female role regarding growing up, completing her schooling, and getting married. She showed an ambivalent dependence upon her mother which is not too unusual. Abby has no friends that she could name. She identifies herself as being a baby and appears to have accepted this role. She was vague about her relationship with her brother and father, except as they might reinforce her baby role. She apparently sees her mother as "wicked," a stimulant of unacceptable anger and not an ego ideal. However, her quotations of her mother and her attempt at presenting herself as a prissy, "good little girl" indicate some desire to fulfill her mother's expectations for her as she understands them.

Comparative Summary

Even without any consideration of the dynamics or the personal and family histories of these two children, it should be obvious that Abby is the sicker of the two youngsters. While the interview does not show Abby to be completely out of contact with reality, conventional reality considerations influence her thinking and behavior much less than is true for Jane. Abby has a breakthrough of primitive instinctual urges. Although she showed less overt and conscious anxiety, her mechanisms of dealing with her feelings appear to be more pathological. Her thinking tends to be tangential, as compared with Jane's, and conversation is stimulated more by her inner fantasies and impulses than by the reality situation. In the area of fantasy Abby reveals much more pathology, both qualitatively and quantitatively. In the area of object relations and identifications Abby appears to be at the level of a much younger child than Jane. There is nothing in either of these interviews to suggest that the girls have any gross impairment of intellect, and this impression was borne out by the formal intellectual assessments previously mentioned.

The mental status observations cannot establish etiology or prognosis beyond question, because behavior is always multidetermined and, like headache or stomach ache, may result from a variety of reasons. However, these data can give clues regarding cause and outcome. Such clues can then be substantiated or refuted by the history and by other physical and psychological testing. There probably is not one specific piece of behavior exhibited by either of these girls which has not been seen at one time or another in other 8-year-olds who were asymptomatic and otherwise functioning satisfactorily.

DYNAMICS OF JANE'S SYMPTOMS. Without the history of the wide discrepancy between intellectual ability and academic achievement in the case of Jane, we are at a loss to be certain whether her over-all maturational process is impaired or not. She showed mild but temporary problems in the affective area. She revealed fears which are commonly a part of growing up, and she is struggling with her dependency relationship with her mother which every human being must do during his maturing years. Projective psychological testing "revealed no sign of psychosis or even any serious neurotic disturbance." We can tentatively postulate that her fears and affective inhibitions may be unusually intense at this time and are interfering with her learning. If so, are her "normal" fears and childish obstinacy being intensified by attitudes and circumstances in the home and/or the school, or is this a temporary reaction to the growth process itself? In brief, Jane appears on examination to have all of the ego functions essential for learning, yet she is not doing so. The only other possible explanation of her school failure is some organically caused specific learning disability. While there was no evidence of gross or "soft" neurological signs during the mental status examination, the possibility of organically determined impairment of learning should be further explored by careful scrutiny of the developmental history and by psychological testing. Further study failed to support any notion of an organic infirmity. However, family history revealed both parents to be shy and inhibited, with a history of problems similar to Jane's in their own school background. Father failed first grade and dropped out at grade ten. Mother completed twelve grades but with great difficulty "due to shyness." They told of sexual and other marital problems about which they do not talk. Both parents stated the mother is overcritical and nagging toward the father, who withdraws into TV viewing. Each claimed to have found some social and vocational satisfaction "by going his own way." They continue to share the same house and the children, yet they find their marriage tolerable rather than satisfying. Both have histories of disrupting relations in their primary families, and neither parent has reached a comfortable emancipation from his own parents. The mother had been moderately punitive with Jane about poor school work and "acting so shy." At the same time she resented the teacher labeling Jane "immature" and felt that psychiatric referral was unnecessary. The diagnostic evaluation concluded that family patterns of interacting and handling emotions are such that these individuals are not realizing their optimum potential in relation to each other and to society. However, they do not suffer any specific psychiatric disease entity. Jane's symptoms are a reaction to the family life. Treatment would have to be directed at improving both intellectual and affective communication among family members. Their repertoire of coping mechanisms would have to be expanded beyond their characteristic patterns of avoidance, denial, withdrawal, and obstinance. In our experience, Jane's school problem should improve with psychotherapy alone and remedial education would not be required. However, if her approach to learning continues beyond the primary grades, treatment will become more complicated.

DYNAMICS OF ABBY'S SYMPTOMS. The disturbance in affect demonstrated by Abby, the second child described, is considered a sign of serious illness. While such a finding could be a temporary reaction to severe stress, the possibility seems unlikely in this case. Abby also shows moderate to marked pathology in her perception of reality, her coping mechanisms, her use of fantasy, her thinking organization, her self concept, and her object relationships. Empirically, we know that this number and degree of ego malfunctions are only seen in seriously ill youngsters whose maturation has been slowed up for a considerable period of time or has been reversed. Psychosis of childhood was the initial diagnostic impression. The causes of the maturational arrest again are not clear from the mental status interview data.

The completed case study, including detailed personal and family histories, physical and neurological evaluations, and psychological testing, confirmed the diagnosis of childhood psychosis. As stated previously, the etiology and dynamics in childhood schizophrenia are unsettled scientific problems. However, in the case of Abby there was overwhelming evidence of a chronic pathological interaction between mother and child since birth. Whether the pathological process began with the mother or child cannot be settled. The pregnancy and birth were described as physically normal, but Abby was "different," more "irritable" and more "difficult," from the beginning. The mother suffered a chronic depression which had existed in a mild to moderate degree for at least five years before Abby's birth. It had been hoped that the new baby might improve the mother's well-being, but her depression and many somatic complaints became worse after the delivery. Throughout infancy and preschool development, the mother-child dyad was characterized by many disappointments and frustrations, with constant battles of will and exchanges of hostility alternating with periods of remorse and intense affection and clinging on the part of both mother and child. The father described himself as a "peace at any price" man who felt helpless to restore equanimity to his home. He was successful in his work and undertook community activities which required him to be away a great deal. He expressed affection toward and interest in Abby but was disappointed and worried. He confirmed his wife's statement that there was some "hard to define" yet definite difference in Abby from the beginning.

EXAMINATION OF AN ADOLESCENT WHO HAS BEEN UNDER CHRONIC STRESS

By the time the child reaches adolescence, it is possible to use the more conventional adult type of interview to assess the patient's mental status. Adolescent patients more nearly fit the standard nosological categories applied to adults than do children. However, young people are still in the process of maturing, and the fluidity of the personality is more like a child's than an adult's. Hence, neurotic syndromes or character disturbances are apt to appear more fleeting and changeable than when such features are present in adults. The adolescent, like the child, is also more vulnerable to environmental stress and is still under the normal pressures of the growing process itself. A "premorbid adjustment" and "specific onset of illness" are harder to define than for adults.

Hence, the degree of developmental impairment is still the *sine qua non* of the severity of illness.

Mental Status Examination

FRED, AGE 14 YEARS. This patient was referred because he "has lost interest in school, going from A's and B's in fifth grade to failure in the seventh." He also has become overtly hostile to his family.

Fred is a tall, slender boy who was dressed in wash pants and sport shirt, like his father. He has bangs down to his eyes, thick glasses, and dental braces. During the initial interview with his parents, Fred kept an almost constant smirk on his face, which would spread to a smile when his various misdeeds were discussed. He appeared quite hostile to both parents, referring to his mother and father as stupid, to his mother as a liar, and to his father as a coward. It was noted that he became anxious only when the interviewer asked about his father's illness. (The father suffers a chronic degenerative hereditary chorea.) In the one-to-one interview he always referred to his parents with defiance and hostility. He avoided showing any remorse or sadness during the four hours he was interviewed. He was friendly and serious with the interviewer but had difficulty maintaining eye contact or showing any emotion other than hostility or self-satisfaction when misconduct was discussed.

The patient was oriented to time, place, and person. No defects in neurosensory perception were noted. Except for a slight slurring of speech, no neurological abnormalities were observed.

His wishes were for a new bike, a go-cart, and a lawn tractor. The patient says he dreams rarely, but when he does they are pleasant dreams about playing with his friends. When asked to draw a picture of a person, he stated that he did not like to draw people and would prefer to draw something else. He did, however, draw a picture of a man whom he described as a beatnik. This beatnik was wearing a shirt with the letters "CSA" on the front, which Fred explained as standing for Confederate States of America. He said, "I was born a Yankee but am a Confederate at heart, and lots of kids are with me too." He saw some clay, asked if he could play with it, and, when told to go ahead, he proceeded to make a cannon "for killing Yankees." Although Fred claimed to have many friends, he had trouble remembering their names. He could not or would not describe activities he enjoys with his friends, and he is not a member of any organized extracurricular groups. Fred fended off any suggestions that he might have problems or be depressed either by total denial or by ignoring the questions. At times he turned his attention completely to reading a newspaper he had brought to the interview. He stated his only problems were trying to get a new bike and one particular teacher at school. He would say such things as "I don't like to think about myself" and when asked why, "Because I'm too busy thinking about riding my bike and playing with my dogs."

Fred responded to every question with concrete answers but never voluntarily started the conversation. He seemed preoccupied with thoughts of weapons and violence and referred to his BB gun and large knife. In a somewhat threatening manner he told the interviewer that he was accurate in throwing his knife up to 60 feet. He also stated that he would like to have a double-barrel shotgun. His favorite play activities are swimming, riding his bike, and fighting. His vocabulary was quite adequate. He spoke matter of factly with no pressure but seemed to take a joy in relating events of violence, e.g., how he punched his sister and shot birds.

Fred appears to have a well-developed intellectual superego in that he readily distinguishes right from wrong. However, when asked about specific misdeeds reported by his parents, he stated that these weren't his fault but were done only for "revenge."

Fred looks at himself as "a little brat." He identifies more closely with his father's illness than with his father, regards himself as "worthless," and thinks in the future he will be a burden to others. He denied much specific knowledge of his father's disease, except that it is hereditary among males. Fred appears to have a high normal IQ.

Even without an item-by-item review of Fred's ego functions, it is apparent that his social and psychological growth is impaired to a moderate degree. His maturation has slowed up to the point where his progress in school and his peer relations are impaired and his relations with his family are deteriorating.

A simple explanation for his school failure might be that his knowledge of a 50-50 chance of impending neurological disease has completely demoralized him. Even his hostility to parents, peers, and the examiner in actions as well as fantasy could be understood as an emotional response to this "impending disaster." If so, this "reaction to stress" gives us a picture of the boy's characteristic defense mechanisms.

Is this character defense specific for chorea or is it a psychological emulation or identification with the father, who was described elsewhere in the case record as being irritable, explosive, and depressed? Depression, irritability, and impaired intellectual functioning have been considered early signs of organic deterioration which may occur several or many years before the onset of the abnormal movements in Huntington's chorea.[55] Questions about specific etiology are thus raised by the mental status exam, but the answers depend upon further study.

It is sufficient for our thesis on the use of the mental status examination to say that this boy shows definite behavioral and personality abnormalities. His disturbance may be the result of either early organic brain disease or functional life-experience factors or both. Not only is he failing to progress socially and intellectually into adolescence, but his ability to cope with feelings of anger and fear seems to be regressing to the preschool level. It is impossible to remove the stress of his reality (the heredity). Therefore, psychological therapy, if it is possible at all, must be directed at reducing fear (possibly through education about this illness), helping him suppress or redirect overt, inappropriate expressions of anger, and improving his self image. Alienating himself from the world as he is now doing may be the only possible outcome for this child's dilemma. However, without a trial of psychotherapy this author cannot accept such a prognosis.

SUMMARY

Mental status profiles for five different children have been presented in detail and their ego functions compared with each other. None of the children showed disturbance in every area of his personality. By qualitative and quantitative assessment of the ego functions, it is possible to estimate the depth of the illness for each child. The mental status examination gives clues regarding etiology and prognosis, but matters pertaining to cause, indicated treatment, and possible outcome must be based upon the total case study, including personal and family history, plus physical and further psychological examinations. In the next sections we will discuss total patient evaluations, of which the mental status examination is only one part.

Chapter 6

NOSOLOGY AND DIAGNOSIS

Hunt, Wittson, and Hunt[38] state that diagnosis is essentially a process of taxonomic categorization with prediction as its function. The accuracy of the prediction will of course depend upon the accuracy of the diagnosis, which in turn implies as thorough knowledge as possible of the causation, the pathogenesis, and the natural course of the illness. An additional function of diagnosis is for professional communication.

The child psychiatrist's examination, the formal mental status evaluation, is only one part of the diagnostic process. Diagnosis involves more than mere "labeling" of the patient's condition. To avoid confusion and misconceptions, one must realize that classificatory terms and diagnoses cannot be used interchangeably. Classification is a problem of nomenclature, while diagnosis has much broader implications.

DIAGNOSTIC CLASSIFICATIONS AND FORMULATIONS

To be correlative with diagnosis, our nomenclature should designate specific types of disorders (symptom complexes), the manner of their development (pathogenesis), their separate causes, and their prognoses. Rutter[61] stresses that a diagnostic classification should convey important and relevant information about the patient, but one should not expect it to say all that is relevant or important. Many clinicians believe that we should use the terms "diagnostic classification" and "diagnostic formulation" separately to avoid compounding our confusion about psychopathology.

The purpose in the development of a scientific nomenclature or categorization is to order our knowledge of childhood psychopathology in such a way that it can be succinctly and accurately communicated to others. The purpose of a "diagnostic formulation" is to provide the basis for a rational treatment approach for one specific child. Classification must be based upon reproducible facts and not upon speculative concepts. Such scientific rigidity is neither possible nor particularly desirable in a diagnostic formulation. The nomenclature is for the classification of disorders, not of children. A diagnostic formulation is for the planning of treatment for a specific child, not for the ordering of childhood disorders.

For many reasons, scientific progress is dependent upon the development of a satisfactory system of classification. As progress is made we would expect the differences between the diagnostic classification of a child's illness and the diagnostic formulation to become less. We would never expect the two concepts to be so identical, however, that we cease treating children with emotional problems and treat only an emotional disorder which happens to have afflicted a child. Classification involves study of the common characteristics of large groups of subjects, while a diagnostic formulation involves the clinical study in depth of an individual patient. Allport[4] has termed the study of groups of subjects the "nomothetic" approach, and the other method the "idiographic" or individual clinical approach.

This author is in sharp disagreement with those who feel that there is little point in distinguishing between different conditions. To be able to understand one's patients, but not to comprehend the language of one's scientific colleagues whose theoretical persuasion differs, seems to be only half fulfillment of professional duty. Indeed, if carried to the extreme, such an attitude will in due course prevent the acquisition of new knowledge and render one comparatively useless to his patients. Some knowledge of the problems of nomenclature seems essential to the understanding of patients and to the meaningful integration of the mental status examination into the diagnostic formulation.

OBSTACLES TO CLASSIFICATION

To date, knowledge about etiology, prognosis, and treatment is insufficient to permit the use of any one of these factors as a common basis for differentiation of mental disorders. Lack of consensus as to pathogenesis is also a problem. The American Psychiatric Association *Diagnostic Manual* of 1952[8] was a giant stride forward for adult psychiatric classification, but it represents only a bare beginning for child psychiatry. As bases for differentiation, the *Manual* uses etiology, prognosis, symptom cluster, severity of disability, and dynamic symptom meaning. Useful though this classification has been, the variability of the basis for the different diagnoses has limited its usefulness for research and epidemiologic studies. Similarly, its clinical usefulness to child psychiatrists leaves much to be desired.

Finch[25] has made some correlations of the American Psychiatric Association categories with current knowledge in child psychopathology. In the American Psychiatric Association Research Report No. 18,[7] several investigators review their attempts at classification which they have found useful both in clinical practice and for research.

Group for the Advancement of Psychiatry Report No. 62, Psychopathological Disorders in Childhood,[33] offers a classification based upon the clinical-descriptive aspects of childhood disorders. Admittedly, such a nomenclature is arbitrary and artificial in many respects. However, this classification does lend itself to statistical tabulation and is employable by psychiatrists of differing theoretical persuasions. In contrast to the G.A.P. classification, the diagnostic formulation outline to be presented in this text is useful only for individual case management and too cumbersome for statistical collecting.

Descriptive classification of mental disorders is especially difficult in child psychiatry because the patient is still a growing, developing organism. The psychic structure remains in a fluid state. Age may color or even be a major determinant in the symptom picture or in the vulnerability to stress.

Etiology is also difficult to incorporate in any classification system. Behavior and thinking are multidetermined. Therefore, in pathologic states multiple causation is the rule, single cause directly related to a specific condition being rare or nonexistent. Different etiologic factors may cause similar symptom pictures; varying symptom complexes may be caused by the same etiologic agents. For example, children with demonstrable brain damage may show thinking and behavior disturbances similar to those in youngsters with no evidence of central nervous system disorder. The structural and physiologic interrelations of the central nervous system have rendered attempts to correlate certain behavior deviations with localized lesions fruitless.

Even when central nervous system abnormalities can be demonstrated, the direct relation of the organic disturbance to specific psychic or behavioral symptoms is often questionable. Children with brain damage frequently show disturbed interpersonal and intrafamily relationships. The question of which is primary and which is secondary may rest more with the theoretical biases of the investigator than with the objective facts. The problem of determining one primary cause is an academic exercise for the psychiatrist. Nevertheless, his conclusions about the relation of pathologic findings to the clinical problems are immediately crucial to treatment planning.

Most youngsters seen in office practice or in child guidance clinics bear no evidence of central nervous system malfunctioning. Careful history-taking will produce ample evidence of disturbed or traumatic relationships and events within the past and present environments to support the thesis of a functional origin. But types of interpersonal relationships and their relation to specific clinical symptoms are not definitively established. In general, the severity of the effect of psychologic trauma is inversely proportional to the age of the child and directly proportional to the duration of the trauma. Yet genetic, constitutional, sociologic, and other variables prevent this latter statement from becoming more than a generalization.

Psychoanalytic theories have been helpful in clarifying some of these relations between events and behavior. Within the analytic context, the relation of ego functioning to past and present relationships and events has become clinically more understandable. Menninger[54] has proposed that many forms of behavior which are termed "symptoms" may be the organism's attempts at restitution or the maintenance of psychologic homeostasis in the face of either internal or external stresses. Some patients may have failed to develop in certain aspects. Others appear to have regressed to more immature mechanisms for coping with either organic or psychic assaults. Such theoretical constructs are extremely useful in planning psychologic therapy or corrective procedures. Nevertheless, the difficulty in establishing direct cause-and-effect relations between events and behavior and the high degree of variability from individual to individual make these constructs extremely difficult to integrate into any system of diagnostic classification. Clinical observation has confirmed that disturbed behavior and many psychic symptoms are reminiscent of or even almost identical with earlier (younger) modes of reacting. In dealing with children, however, the matter of age-appropriateness for various behaviors is subject to clinical judgment and much debate.

Anna Freud[27] describes an interesting obstacle to any definitive classification of mental disorders in children. She points out that temporary ego regressions are a part of normal child development. They may be a reaction to everyday stresses of tiredness, anxiety of separation, or physical illness. In addition, the growth process itself broadens the child's reality awareness and exposes him to many painful and anxiety-provoking aspects of life. Miss Freud's thesis is a confirmation of the fact that no child's development progresses along a steady linear course, but that children take two steps forward and one step backward. Such regressions appear to be beneficial if they are temporary and spontaneously reversible. Prolongation of regression may result in disturbances of relationships and become a pathogenic agent in itself. The situation is further complicated by the difficulty in differentiating temporary from more permanent regressions and accurately predicting a spontaneous return to previous levels of adjustment. Parents give recognition to this phenomenon when they ask, "Is he emotionally ill or is he just going through a stage?"

THE DIAGNOSTIC FORMULATION

Difficult though diagnostic classification may be, the clinician need not despair of helping his patient. He can develop a diagnostic formulation and rational treatment plan based upon knowledge of the individual patient and the accumulated body of theory and facts about childhood emotional disorders. Our concept of diagnostic formulation is similar to what Menninger[53] has termed "diagnostic synthesis," and the "Dynamic Genetic Formulation" outline in the Appendix of G.A.P. Report No. 62.[33] Detailed comprehension of the multiple determinants of individual personality functioning is vital to intelligent clinical management.

The clinician must be familiar with the literature and have had some clinical psychiatric experience in order to participate in either diagnostic or therapeutic work with children. Comprehension of the diagnostic formulation requires some understanding of sociomedical history-taking and the multidisciplinary team approach which have been the *modus operandi* of clinical child psychiatry for the past thirty-five to forty years. The beginner is urged to read Report No. 38 of the Group for the Advancement of Psychiatry[32] for a brief review of long-accepted practices in child guidance clinics. This author will also review here a case history outline and case material to demonstrate the integration of data about the physical, emotional, and social aspects of the past and present life of the child into a formulation and treatment plan.

The diagnostic formulation and treatment plan contain the answers, so far as these are possible, to eight implicit questions:

1. How sick or impaired is this child?
2. In what areas of his functioning is the impairment manifested, and in what areas does he function well? (See Outline for Mental Status Examination of a Child, page 51.)
3. Is there any past or present evidence that the central nervous system is not functionally intact?
4. What psychosocial factors in his past life have probably contributed to the problem?
5. Which psychosocial factors in his current life continue to contribute to his problem or are apt to be an impediment to recovery?
6. Which of the factors under questions 2, 3, 4, and 5 is it imperative to change in order for improvement to occur?
7. Which factors under questions 2, 3, 4, and 5 would the clinician desire to change for the general well-being of the child, although perhaps not essential for change in the child's presenting symptoms?
8. What methods, if any, can be used to effect the desired changes noted under questions 6 and 7?

All these questions are related to three basic issues: in what manner is this child's functioning impaired, why is this so, and what can be done about it? These questions do not separate easily. This difficulty in separating cause and effect may explain why some centers tend to treat all children with a "shotgun" therapeutic approach or why the work of other centers seems to confirm and reinforce preconceived theories about the major causes and most effective treatment approaches to most childhood emotional problems. The foregoing eight-item breakdown in the diagnostic formulation considers the fact that there are usually multiple impairments and multiple causes. Empirically, prognosis seems to have a direct quantitative relation to questions 1 through 5. Although qualitative factors also play a role in prognosis, the greater the number of disturbed ego functions (question 2) and the greater the number of apparent contributing causes (questions 3, 4, and 5), the worse the outlook seems to be.

In our experience the most severely impaired children, generally termed psychotic, show moderate to severe deviations in all or nearly all the items listed in the mental status examination (page 35). The prognosis is uniformly guarded for all of these children. It is commonly assumed that psychotic children with demonstrable central nervous system pathology have an even worse prognosis than those with no organic impairment. Nevertheless a child with a neurologic impairment may have a considerably better chance of at least social recovery than a child with a severly disturbed psychosocial environment. Actually, a child with both impairment of brain functioning and a problematic situation in his environment may have the least chance of all for attaining reasonably normal adjustment levels.

A low number and mild degree of ego deviations (question 2) do not necessarily indicate that the child will spontaneously improve or be treated easily. A child with severe anxiety who displays many neurotic defense mechanisms may respond well to outpatient psychotherapy, provided he has a reasonably intact superego, demonstrates the capacity for meaningful interpersonal relations (see question 2), and his family members are relatively free of unchangeable neurotic interaction patterns which perpetuate his problems (see question 5). A great difference in the answers to questions 2 and 5 for a particular child could alter the situation to the extent that outpatient psychotherapy alone would not be sufficient to help him.

The number of possible answers to each of the foregoing eight questions and the number of possible combinations of answers make it impractical to outline absolute rules for treatment programming or prognostication in every conceivable type of case. Diagnosis and treatment depend upon clinical experience and judgment. The information gathered from the psychiatrist's examination, supplemented by social history and psychologic data, should provide answers to the first three questions. The detailed social history and evaluation of the parents will supply answers to questions 5 and 6. On the basis of the total information, treatment planning and prognosis are based.

SUMMARY

Diagnostic classification of childhood mental disorders and the diagnostic formulation of a particular child's disability are two somewhat overlapping tasks of child psychiatrists which have distinctly different objectives. Classification serves to organize the accumulated body of knowledge of the psychopathology of childhood for the clinician and the scientific investigator. Formulation of a specific child's disability serves as a rational basis for designing a treatment plan for that child. The former is a nomothetic approach, the latter idiographic. We must strive for knowledge that will make classification and diagnostic formulations similar and complementary to each other. It is neither possible nor desirable, however, at this time to make these two clinical, scientific functions identical in process or aim.

A diagnostic formulation outline consisting of eight questions has been offered. Several of these questions can be answered only by history and by examination of significant elements of the child's environment. History-taking,[32,34] family dynamics,[1,39,42,77] and child neurology[22,43,51] are reviewed elsewhere in the literature.

The first four chapters of this text discussed the child's mental status examination, a procedure which seems to us to have been comparatively neglected in the literature. We will now briefly review history-taking and demonstrate how the history, psychological testing, and mental status examination may be integrated into a complete case study and diagnostic formulation.

Chapter 7

INTERVIEWING THE PARENTS

Obtaining the history of the patient has been an accepted practice for so long that any questions about it or review of its content may seem to be unnecessary. Even so, the history of the child psychiatric patient has such special significance that it deserves separate consideration.

The direct psychiatric examination of the child has been discussed in detail first in this monograph to underscore its importance. However, as stated in earlier sections, certain facts essential for diagnosis and treatment planning can only be obtained from the parents. These particulars, essentially unknown to the child, are his early development, past physical and psychological stresses, a comparison of his social-developmental level with his age group, characteristics of the parental relationship, and an objective assessment of the emotional well-being of each parent.

TWO DISPARATE ATTITUDES

The approach to the parents can be considered from two extreme but inaccurate points of view. One position is that the parents are without a doubt the direct cause of the child's symptoms. Any information to the contrary arises merely from parental resistance to accepting the blame and taking corrective measures. The opposite stance is that parents have unjustifiably been made scapegoats by child development theorists. In this view, children's symptoms are seen as the result of some quirk of fate, "bad seed," or elusive organic central nervous system impairment. Hence, parents are interviewed for the sole purpose of obtaining an "objective" history of the child's symptoms and development. Those with this latter attitude toward parents consider the emotional interplay within the family irrelevant. Some students readily sympathize with cooperative, poised, interested parents who share the student's own value system. However, they make whipping boys of parents who are inarticulate or whose views on race, religion, politics, sex, child rearing, and other sociocultural phenomena are different from the interviewer's own position.

The behavioral scientist or serious student of human behavior strives for objectivity and takes pride in any success he may achieve in freeing himself of biases. Even so, it is often impossible to know whether certain parental attitudes or practices are truly pathogenic or are merely called deviant because they are distasteful or incomprehensible to the investigator. Sears and associates[64] document the great variety of childhood experiences evident among American children of a similar sociocultural economic class and the tremendous task of relating these experiences to specific aspects of each child's personality. Clinical experience, research, and common sense tell us that every parent influences the behavior and development of his child in an infinite number of ways. Even so, we must await much more extensive basic research in the behavioral sciences before we can completely understand the complicated interplay between the environmental experiences and the genetic-constitutional endowment of the child which underlie each symptom complex.

At least current knowledge and practices have made the old game of either condemning or exonerating parents as passé as the controversy of organic versus functional etiology. In some cases, parental attitudes and behavior will be highly relevant to the child's problems. In other cases, circumstances of fate or the child's native personality endowment will be more important. In still other situations, a complicated admixture of the child's temperament and his life experiences will be the only logical explanation for his symptom picture.

To achieve an accurate and useful diagnostic formulation, the clinician must maintain the same sympathetic, inquisitive approach to the parents that he has toward the child. By conscientiously trying to obtain an impression of both the assets and liabilities of each parent's personality and their relationship with each other and with their child, the interviewer should be able to prevent his own value judgments from distorting the interview process.

Premature efforts to differentiate "normal" and "pathological" parental behavior should be avoided. Such "good" and "bad" judgments on isolated bits of behavior are likely to reflect the clinician's feelings about his own upbringing and have only incidental relevance to the problems presented by his patient. Zuckerman,[75,76] Mark,[49] Shoben,[65] Becker,[11] and others have attempted to use consciously stated parental attitudes to differentiate parents of normal children from parents of maladjusted children without success. Gildea and her associates[23] found little relationship between specific parental attitudes and adjustment in a group of school children. However they did feel there were significant relationships between "patterns of attitude combinations and adjustment." The interviewer needs to know each parent's attitude and the effective experiences associated with the pregnancy and birth. When and how the child was fed, trained, disciplined, loved, and taught about property rights, sex, and so on, are all important. However, it is the total shape or arrangement of the parent-child interaction which is important to his development. Isolated events which the parents can tell you or which can be observed, together with understanding of the parents' strengths and weaknesses, must be woven into patterns which portray the daily emotional life of the child. On the basis of their longitudinal study of 136 children for more than ten years, Chess and her associates[19] also conclude that "parent-child interaction should be analyzed not only for parental influences on the child but just as much for the influence of the child's individual characteristics on the parent."

INTERVIEWING VERSUS HISTORY-TAKING

We have called this chapter "Interviewing the Parents" in preference to "History-taking" because of the broader implication of the term "interview." It is essential to have a historical account of the child's presenting problems, the course of symptoms, his current over-all adjustment, and his past physical and psychological development from conception to the present time. However, we also need data about the past and present emotional climate of the home and an assessment of the physical and mental health of each parent. These data are not only important to etiology and diagnosis but should be highly influential in determining the choice of treatment and the prognosis. The natural dependency of the child makes the parent an essential party to his treatment as well as to his pathology.

In a recent publication[67] the author has reviewed methods for sociomedical-psychological history-taking in a pediatric outpatient clinic. The same principles apply to the history of a child with an identifiable emotional problem. A noncondemning, fact-gathering approach helps to lessen parental guardedness and defensiveness. To enhance the accuracy of the history and to obtain the maximum parental cooperation, the necessity of interviews with each parent by oneself or by a member of one's own staff cannot be overemphasized.

Helper[36] and Levitt[46] have found low agreement between children's self-evaluations and evaluations of them by their parents. Clinically, it is often evident that each parent has quite different ideas about their child and each other. It is, therefore, quite important to review the salient points of the history in a family group interview and to see the parents together without the child as well as to interview each parent alone. When the child lives full or part-time with both parents, direct interviews with each of them is necessary for an accurate history. The old practice of seeing only mother and child has been discarded in favor of interviewing the mother-father-child triad or even including entire families in the diagnosis and treatment. The subtle interaction patterns which constitute family relationships cannot be comprehended without firsthand acquaintance with all of the principals.

An outline for recording the child's and the family's history follows. In addition, the examiner needs to know something of each parent's personal adjustment and reaction patterns within the family. It could be said that we need to have a mental status examination of each parent. However, a comparatively brief, personal sociomedical-psychological history is probably more palatable to the parents and more accurately reflects current practices. This is an abbreviated list of topics and questions to be discussed in the parent interviews. Of course, the parents should not be vigorously interrogated on each of these subjects. They should be permitted to tell their story spontaneously in their own manner. The interviewer should guide the discussion in order that the various topics are covered in whatever order the parents' comfort indicates.

OUTLINE FOR INTERVIEWING THE PARENTS

1. Child's history
   a. Parents' main concerns about the child (chief complaint or presenting problem)
   b. Course of symptoms and current adjustment
   c. Past developmental, medical, social, and psychological history, including peer and school adjustments
   d. Child's relationships with siblings and each parent
2. Parents' marital history
3. Parents' personal history
   a. Parents' primary family, past and present
   b. School and vocational adjustment
   c. Social and avocational interests and activities
   d. Review of any specific medical or psychological problems suffered by either parent
4. Other family problems (other children, previous marriages, in-laws, neighbors, etc.)

5. Parents' opinions about possible causes, and a review of their feelings about various treatments that might be proposed

Child's History

Most parents are defensive about their child. The defensiveness and guardedness will be enhanced if the parent is asked to tell what's "wrong" or what he "thinks" is wrong with the child. Words like "wrong," "bad," "problem," and "trouble" are best avoided. An invitation to *describe* or tell about the child gives unspoken recognition of normal parental ambivalence and encourages the parent to state both his positive and negative views of the child's adjustment. Many parents very easily and spontaneously give a full history of the child with little prodding or direction from the interviewer. If the parent seems to be at a loss for words or to be holding back information, questions regarding dates and circumstances of significant events or developmental milestones can help to get him started talking. As he relaxes, inquiry can then be made into emotionally charged symptoms or events if these facts are not spontaneously related.

Each parent's knowledge of the child and family lies in three levels of his consciousness. First, there are facts and opinions which are in his foreconscious and which he will readily tell to most anyone. Secondly, there are certain things which he consciously withholds from the interviewer because of distrust, fear of embarrassment, or because he does not consider them relevant to the examination. Finally, there is a wealth of valuable data which the parent has repressed or forgotten because of its emotional charge. If the interviewer-parent relationship promotes trust and is skillfully directed, the parent will voluntarily reveal more and more about himself and the family. This process in turn stimulates associations and often releases repressed material. Frequently, parents are surprised themselves at the many forgotten but significant events which come to their minds as a result of the interviews. Of course, much important repressed material cannot be released during diagnosis but must await therapy when indicated.

If the suggestions given do not facilitate the parent's verbal productivity, it can be assumed that the cause of the reticence lies with something outside the immediate interviewer-parent relationship. Paucity of words may be merely a personality characteristic of the parent, and nothing can be done but record it as an observation. Frequently, though, defensiveness is caused by feelings of shame or anger or the circumstances surrounding the referral. Inquiry into the parent's concept of the child's or family's need for help should bring out these feelings. Often it is necessary to permit the parent to spend considerable time ventilating his anger about the referring individual or agency before he can give the child's history.

Mr. R. appeared impatient and irritable. He did not talk spontaneously. When asked to tell his reasons for bringing his son, Mike, for examination he replied, "They say he has a school problem." In response to the query of what Mr. R. considered Mike's school problem to be, he said, "He [apparently meaning the teacher or principal] said Mike acted up in class, disturbed the other kids, and last week pushed a boy down the steps. I don't know what's wrong over at that school, but we don't have trouble like that around home. The schools today don't even try to have good discipline." The interviewer commented that the family must be pretty annoyed to have Mike sent for examination with false accusations. Mr. R. responded that the allegations may have been partially true but he resented Mike being singled out. The school certainly had plenty of children whose behavior was worse. He then launched into a lengthy discussion of the school's discrimination against laboring-class families. There were plenty of rumors about the principal being incompetent and possibly immoral. Many parents are ready to expose the fact that most of the teachers are unfit for their jobs. After considerable ventilation, Mr. R. stated that Mike had probably done those things, but "He is not a mental case." His mother couldn't handle him, but that was her fault. Mr. R. had repeatedly told her to crack down. She was always tired out and depressed. She babied the boy and then complained to him. "Mike is no mental case." He knew better. He never acted that way when the father was home. "I won't stand for it. The school and his mother ought to thrash him. I've told them to."

Having released much feeling, Mr. R. was then able to give other information about his child and family fairly easily.

Parents' Marital History

The marital relationship is a very private and sensitive topic which must be approached forthrightly but with tact and discretion. This subject might be introduced by a statement that many parents are surprised and embarrassed that we ask personal questions about their relationship with their marital partner. However, in the interest of helping us understand their child, we hope they will answer such questions to the best of their ability. Such a direct request for cooperation is reassuring to the parents and is seldom refused by them. Some discuss their associations with their spouses readily. Whether they do so easily or not, it is important to know the length of courtship, ages at the time of marriage, reactions of family to the marriage, type of family planning if any, and who has assumed the dominant role regarding money, decisions, child discipline, the sexual adjustment, etc. What was the reason for the marriage? This may be approached by inquiry into what attracted the parents to each other. The romantic idea of intense, irresistible love is probably responsible for much less than half the marriages. Frequently, marital discontent is due to unfulfilled fantasies about what the marriage should be, even though these wishes or hopes were never verbalized even to the self. Multiple marriages and separations for any reason must be inquired about. Often the diagnostic inquiry brings about the parent's first reflection on the child's reactions to such events.

Parents' Personal History and Attitudes toward Treatment

Individuals who can talk about the foregoing topics usually have little difficulty giving their own personal history. The simple explanation should be given that it will help in the understanding of the patient if we know something of each parent's primary family and upbringing. The interviewer cannot be satisfied with the statement that "my own childhood was normal" without knowing the informant's concept of normalcy. The culture, the early relationships, and events which have influenced the mother's or father's attitudes and behavior about parenthood are important to know.

Specific treatment recommendations cannot be made until the study is completed. Nevertheless, some preliminary discussion of the family's reactions to various possible treatment plans have both therapeutic and prognostic value. Previous treatments and corrective procedures considered by the parents should be reviewed. The most frequently made recommendation for child psychiatric problems are individual psychotherapy for one or more members of the family, group therapy, conjoint therapy, family group therapy, tutoring and remedial education, or environmental manipulations such as adjustments of school curriculum, change of schools, boarding school, residential treatment school, or hospital. The treatment possibilities most likely for the case in hand should be explained to the parents. Their response will often reveal the degree to which they understand the child's symptoms and the degree to which they personally are able or willing to participate in treatment. In addition, pragmatic issues such as cost, frequency of visits, length of treatment, distance of home from treatment center, and availability of community resources nearer their home all have a direct bearing on parental acceptance of the final recommendations and are significant for prognostication.

Levitt[47] postulated that expectation-reality discrepancy (ERD) is negatively related to favorable therapy outcome. He suggests that education of the patient (and parent) about his role in treatment should be done. Reduction of the difference between the patient's expectations of what therapy will be like and what really will occur can have a "catalytic effect" on treatment outcome. Simply stated, it seems reasonable that a good rational, intellectual grasp of various corrective procedures is essential for maxium parental cooperation. Hence, a systematic review of various forms of treatment is needed to give the parents some intellectual understanding of the various types of corrective procedures which may be recommended for their child.

SUMMARY

In this book we have emphasized the importance of directly interviewing the child patient, feeling that in the literature and in practice there has been too much reliance on the history as given by the parent and too little attention paid to careful examination of the child. However, we do not intend to minimize or overlook the importance of a careful history from the parents. This chapter has reviewed some general principles regarding parent interviews.

The clinician must avoid blaming the parent for all of the child's problems. On the other hand he should not overlook the fact that parental personalities and family events are relevant to the child's personality development. To obtain accurate historical data and to comprehend the subtle family interaction patterns, both parents should be included in the diagnostic study. Mother and father should be interviewed in the presence of their child, with each other in the absence of the child, and individually. These series of interviews should cover: (1) the child's complete personal history, (2) the parents' marital history, (3) personal and family history of each parent, (4) the family culture, and (5) parental attitudes about causes and possible approaches to (remedial) treatment.

Basic knowledge of parents and family assists in understanding the dynamics of the child's illness. Family personalities and events are not always the cause of the symptoms, but they are always essential elements in treatment and prognosis. The development of symptoms usually disrupts important interhuman relations, and disturbed relationships are often the cause of symptoms. Hence, many families at the time of examination have a self-feeding pathological interaction system established. The natural dependency of the child makes his parents the most significant part of his environment. To attempt to diagnose or treat the child without the assistance of his parents or parent substitutes would be like trying to create a psychological vacuum.

Chapter 8

THE CASE STUDY

A COMPLETE case study will contain a past and present history of the child, a family history and an assessment of significant members of the child's current household, the psychological test results, and the mental status report. A summation of these data should permit the clinical team or the individual clinician to make a diagnostic formulation and treatment plan for a particular child.

Some case material will be presented to illustrate how our case study method leads to a diagnostic formulation. The formulation reflects the clinician's opinions regarding the type and severity of the emotional disorder, the most probable causes and contributing factors, and what he feels is the best course of treatment for the patient. Admittedly, treatment is strongly influenced by the theoretical orientation of the clinician. Even so, theoretical constructs have to be adapted to the specific variety of disorder presented by the patient. The selection of which treatment for which child is dependent upon clinical judgment. Clinical acumen is continually influenced by the rapidly expanding body of knowledge regarding etiology and treatment methods.

In Chapter 6 the diagnostic formulation was defined as containing answers to the eight implicit questions appearing on p. 110. These questions guide the examiner in outlining the seriousness of the illness, the cause or causes, the treatment, and the prognosis.

Neither the history, the psychological testing, nor the psychiatric examination alone can provide all of the answers to these questions. The history from the parents or guardians and the school will give the parents' and teachers' views of the types and severity of impairments which they see in the child. The degree of illness and areas of relative health or impairment in the child's personality will be more specifically identified by the psychologist's and psychiatrist's reports. Evidence for central nervous system impairment (question 3) will be obtained from the history of birth, development, systems review, and past illnesses, from the physical and neurological findings, and from the impressions of the psychologist and psychiatrist. The relevance of these findings to the presenting symptoms and personality configurations rests with clinical judgment. In a similar fashion, conclusions about the presence and relative importance of psychosocial factors will be drawn from the history and from direct examinations, evaluated in the context of the clinician's current knowledge and hypotheses regarding psychopathogenesis.

The practice of establishing *either* a functional *or* an organic etiology has become passé. As diagnostic acumen has developed, clinicians are finding more and more cases in which both organic and functional factors appear to have been significant in the development of a particular disturbance. One or the other of these factors alone would either have not resulted in the development of disordered adjustment or would have resulted in a different symptom complex.

Similarly, as stated in Chapter 6, child psychiatrists have broadened their concept of functional etiology beyond the premise of the disturbed mother-child relationship. Experience has taught that father-child relationships, mother-father interaction, or entire family interactions are significant. Cultural and economic phenomena cannot be ignored because of their influence on the configuration of family interaction patterns.

Multiple etiology is at least theoretically possible in every case and glaringly apparent in many. With this tenet the "either-or" concept of etiology is not very helpful clinically. The clinical questions are summarized in questions 6 and 7: How have the most probable causes converged to produce the symptom picture? Which of these contributing causes are still active and problematic to the situation? The answer to these questions leads to the final question of what can and must be done in the way of corrective procedures?

A diagnostic-treatment model can be illustrated by comparing child psychiatric treatment to some aspects of orthopedic surgery. The surgeon never "cures" a broken bone. He approximates the fragments and then places the injured part in a highly protective environment, the cast, to prevent further trauma or noxious agents from influencing the healing process. If the bone pathology is too severe or if healing fails to take place with conservative measures, he must then probe deeply into the seat of the pathology and attempt to make structural and other changes. At the risk of oversimplification, psychiatric treatment of children can be seen as an attempt insofar as possible to remove noxious and traumatic agents to permit healthy development to take place. Often psychotherapeutic effort to change ideas, feelings, and neurotic concepts is necessary in one or more members of the family. Whenever psychotherapy is used, concomitant manipulation of the immediate environment and a gradual resumption of normal functioning are always essential aspects of treatment. Injured bones and injured personalities never heal without scarring and some functional impairment. The ultimate goal of treatment is to achieve minimal disability. Successful treatment never provides insurance against future breaks under sufficient stress, but future problems can often be reduced if the degree of fragility of the organism is fully understood.

The case study outline on the next few pages permits summarization of the evaluation data, yet is sufficiently inclusive and flexible to be applicable to a wide variety of conditions. The outline can be used to record the summary of relatively uncomplicated cases as well as to summarize the important information about children with multiple problems due to a diversity of causes.

Outline for Case Study*

1. *Identifying Data:*

Name: _____ Case No.: _____

Address: _____ Intake Date: _____

Tel. No.: _____ Race: _____ Birth Date: _____ Age: _____

School: _____ Grade: _____

Religion: _____ Referred By: _____

Current Family	Name	Relation to Patient	Age	Occupation or Grade
Father				
Mother				
Children (Including Patient)				

Natural Parents	Deceased Family Members (Relation to Patient)	Date
Married		
Separated		
Divorced		

---

*From Green, Morris and Haggery, Robert J.: *Ambulatory Pediatrics*. Philadelphia, W. B. Saunders Company, 1968, with permission of authors and publisher.

2. *Presenting Problem:*

3. *Course of Symptoms and Current Adjustment of Child: (Present illness):*

4. *Family Picture:*

5. *Preschool Developmental History* (Includes prenatal history):

6. *Medical History* (Includes systems review plus past illnesses, injuries and operations):

7. *School History:*

8. *Mother* (Personal history):

9. *Father* (Personal history):

10. *Child:*
   A. Mental Status Examination
   B. Physical Examination
   C. Special Procedures
      1. Laboratory
      2. Psychological test results
      3. Consultation results

11. *Diagnostic Formulation:*
   A. The major symptoms or problems as discerned from both history and direct observations.
   B. The physical, emotional, and social (including family) factors which have caused or are contributing to the symptoms.
   C. Treatment given or planned

12. *Follow-up Visits* (Including parental conferences):

13. *Treatment Reviews:*
   A. Current working formulation and progress
      1. The child
      2. The parents
   B. Recommendations for further treatment

On the following pages, three cases are presented in detail. The average clinician is confronted with a wide variety of psychiatric problems. The outline method of recording clinical data serves as a guide for the clinical case study and illustrates the process of case analysis and synthesis which is essential to treatment planning.

REFUSAL TO ATTEND SCHOOL (SCHOOL PHOBIA)

Name: Jeffrey M.

Birth Date: 8-29-59   Age: 6½ years

School: Consolidated Elementary

Religion: Protestant

Referred By: Family physician, Dr. N. B.

Family		Relation to Patient	Age	Occupation or Grade
Father	R.M.	Father	42	Machinist
Mother	E.M.	Mother	35	Housewife
Children	F.M.	Sister	12	Sixth grade
	G.M.	Brother	10	Fourth grade
	J.M.	Patient	6½	First grade

Deceased Family Members:

Paternal grandfather died in 1940 at age 65
Maternal grandmother died in the fall of 1965
at age 65

Presenting Problem:

"He doesn't want to go to school." Since the
death of his maternal grandmother four months
ago, Jeff has not wanted to go to school. When he
was sent to school, he just sat in his seat and
cried for two hours or so until his parents were
asked to come and take him home. If anyone tried
to get him to work, he would become sassy. At
home he is usually a very good boy, and the
mother says, "He is a comfort to me because I
need someone in the house with me." Only when an

attempt is made to separate him from his mother does he become stubborn and angry.

Course of Symptoms and Current Adjustment of Child:

Jeff started the first grade in September of 1965 at age six. Both his mother and the school principal state he was doing quite well and seemed to like school. In November Jeff contracted the measles. While he was home, the news came that Mrs. M's mother had died suddenly. Neither Jeff nor the other children seemed to be unduly disturbed by the news of their grandmother's death. The mother took it very hard and broke down and cried openly and frequently. By the time of the funeral, Jeff was almost well from the measles but was kept home from school another week. During this time the mother made daily trips to MGM's grave and took Jeff with her. When Jeff was again sent back to school, he said he didn't want to go and upon arrival there just sat in his seat and cried. He told the teacher and his parents that he was afraid to go away from home because he thought his mother might not be there when he came back.

After a week or two of this behavior, he was removed from school on the advice of Dr. S. While at home with his mother, the daily trips to the MGM's grave were continued. The mother also consulted Dr. B., who told her to stop the daily trips to the grave and prescribed some nerve pills for her and a white nerve medicine for Jeff. Mrs. M. says that the nerve pills help her to some extent when she takes them, but that for quite a while Jeff would take his nerve medicine and spit it out in the bathroom. During this time she states that he was quite nervous and upset. He would jump up and down and shake all over in excitement but apparently enjoyed watching some TV programs (such as "Leave It to Beaver"). When she discovered he was not swallowing his nerve medicine, she forced him to swallow it in front of her and he became calmer. Mrs. M. was advised by her physician to try to wean Jeff from his dependence upon her by leaving him with friends for a few minutes at a time and by starting him into school a few minutes each day and increasing this time until he could stay there all day. She had little success with this program, however, and the boy has not gone back to school.

Jeff has continued to enjoy playing with his brother and sister and to go to church and Sunday school with the family. Mrs. M. thinks that his behavior is improving slightly and that she herself is beginning to feel better in accepting her mother's death.

Background Information

Family Picture:

The family lives in a modern three-bedroom home built by the father in a rural area. The boys share one bedroom, each with his own bed, and the parents and sister have the other two. The two older children have continued in school and are seemingly unaffected by the present problem. The marriage has been generally harmonious with mutual discussion of problems and plans. The mother is dissatisfied with the marriage in that she would desire to have sexual relations more than once a week. She feels her husband is inconsiderate in frequently forgetting to give her birthday, anniversary, and

Christmas gifts. Their monthly payments for house, furniture, and car burden them so that she cannot afford to buy a set of false teeth. The MGPs have lived nearby, and Mrs. M. has often been called upon to help them out when they were not feeling well. She also does cleaning work at their church and takes in ironing for pay in order to help supplement the family income and to keep herself busy.

Preschool Developmental History:

Except for slight nausea and vomiting during the first two months, the pregnancy was normal until the last two months, when Mrs. M. states that she became so big that she could hardly walk because of pressure and pains down below. He was born two weeks late, weighing 8 pounds, 13½ ounces (2 pounds more than the other two children), after a nine-hour labor during which the pains were harder and quicker than those during the other pregnancies. The mother was given gas for the delivery and was told that he was born head first and everything was normal. Mother and child left the hospital the second day after birth, and she began to nurse him. She believes her milk was not rich enough because he nursed all the time and she thought he was losing weight although he was not weighed. After one week of nursing he was changed to SMA formula, which he vomited, and then to Wilson formula, which he vomited, and finally when he was 10 days old she put him on straight homogenized milk, which agreed with him and he thrived thereafter. Mother absolutely cannot recall when he sat up, walked, or began to talk, although she thinks these were at normal intervals. She states that he cried more than her other children, especially when she would leave the room or the house. Toilet training was started about two years of age, and it took only a few months to accomplish this. He has not been enuretic or incontinent since.

School History:

See Course of Symptoms

Medical History:

He has had all immunizations. Had frequent respiratory infections until a year ago and measles in November of last year.

Mother:

Mrs. M. is a plainly dressed woman of 35 who looks more like 50. She has a very sad expression on her face, no teeth, and readily talks of how sad she is and of how she believes that her friends and even her own sister do not care for her. She is the fifth in a family of eight children. She describes MGF as a good man who was strict and trained the children well. He was a farmer and also worked on the railroad section crew and did carpentry work on the side. He did not go to church with the family or to other activities with the children. She describes MGM as being a good woman, always giving to others (although not sacrificing her own needs). She took the children to church and was very happy when they joined. The youngest child, Ellen, now 21, was her favorite. Ellen was born during the time when MGM was "in the change of life" and has always been sickly, having trouble with her stomach and nerves. All the mother's siblings except Ellen quit school because they didn't like it or to get married. Only Ellen completed high school. Mrs. M. herself had to drop out of school at the age of 16 after completing the eighth grade in order to take care of MGM. MGM had been an ambitious, hard-working woman who liked to have large crowds of company, as many as fifty at a time. She was also sickly with "rheumatism and arthritis"; when Mrs. M. was 16 these became so bad that she had to use crutches and a cane for about six months. Doctoring with home remedies such as lemon juice helped MGM become well enough to get rid of the crutches and cane. In spite of this, the mother still remained at home until she met her husband and married at the age of 19.

Mrs. M. has always been sensitive to criticism and even in the first grade would cry if scolded by the teacher. She has always regretted that she couldn't finish high school. She looks back on her childhood in the country and says that "life was better then than life is now." When her brother died in 1943, MGM had a "heart attack" and was sick in bed with trouble breathing for a week but did not go to the hospital.

The mother's description of meeting the father is as he gave it. She says that she was attracted to him because he was not smart or flirty like some boys. He didn't drink. He was good-looking and a steady worker. She says that she wanted four children but does not state a preference as to sex. She has enjoyed their sexual relations and achieves a climax each time. Though she wanted to have four children, the doctor told her that it would be too hard on her to have any more because Jeff had been so big that he had injured her too badly to allow her to have another child. After Jeff was born, they moved to their present house, which seemed too big to keep clean. She became afraid to whip and discipline the children because she thought she might hurt them. During this time she also cried a lot and was given some nerve pills, which she took for a month or two. She feels very gloomy and blue for a couple of days before each period. About four years ago she went through several months during which she had cramping low abdominal pains prior to each menstrual period, and exploratory surgery was performed. Her appendix was removed, and she was told that she had pinworms in it. A cyst was also removed from one ovary, though the doctor said there was no danger from this. She has not had abdominal pain since.

The mother says that she has again begun to cry more during the past year. She has also felt that their friends and even her sister do not really care for her, and has felt more acutely her husband's neglect of anniversaries and birthdays. She was quite grieved by the death of her mother and says it was a comfort to have Jeff home with her. On the other hand, she feels that if he had not been home with the measles the first week after her mother's death that she would have been able to "work out my problems better myself." She does cleaning work at her church and also takes in ironing, stating she would "rather iron than eat."

About June or July of 1965 (ten months ago)

she had a severe headache from "sinus trouble." She told her sister that "if I did not think it would make people talk I would just take this whole bottle of Anacin to get rid of my troubles." She feels that life is not worth living, that she would just like to go to bed and get away from it all and cry all day, but other than that one instance she has not thought of suicide. She sleeps well and has no trouble going to sleep at night or waking up in the middle of the night. About two years ago she had one bad dream which she blames on her nerves. She felt all the walls of the room were closing in on her and she couldn't escape. She also worries about family finances. She feels that she takes everybody's worries on herself.

Mrs. M's insight into her own and Jeff's problems is slight, though by the second interview she stated that perhaps the problem might be her "nerves" and not just Jeff's being stubborn and not wanting to go to school. It is the examiner's impression that mother is a rather dependent person, always closely tied to MGM, striving to please her and other authority figures, having sacrificed her education for her mother and suffering rivalry with the favored younger sister. She seems to be moderately depressed at this time and has shown symptoms of depression ever since Jeff's birth.

Father:

Mr. M., age 42, is the youngest in a family of six, including two half siblings by a former marriage of his mother. He is a plain man dressed in working clothes who states that he does not like to come to Metropolis because he always gets lost in the big city. (On visits to the clinic the family is brought by a sister of Mrs. M. who lives in the suburbs and drives them across the city.) PGF is described as a "typical old farmer" who barely made enough to get by on a twenty-acre farm in spite of being a very hard worker. He was described as very kindhearted. He was relatively easygoing in comparison to PGM but was able to keep law and order among the children by use of a razor strap or belt. PGM is described as the one who had the drive in the family. PGM took all the children to church every week, though PGF seldom went. The father cannot describe any particular closeness to either one of his parents.

Mr. M. seems to have had a relatively uneventful boyhood, riding horses, playing ball, going hunting, going on hay rides with the young people from the church, and attending movies for entertainment. Of course, he had to work hard on the farm as well. He enjoyed school and made fairly good grades. He took all the courses in Latin offered at his school and wanted to go on to further courses but could not because they did not teach them. During his junior year in high school his father died of kidney trouble, and the next spring he had to quit school and get a job "in order to have enough to eat." His two full sisters who are just a few years older than he were able to complete high school. He went to work as a farm hand and had various jobs until called into the army near the end of the Second World War. He completed training just in time to spend eighteen months in the Army of Occupation as an MP. He went around with some of the German girls but "did not do the things that many of the other soldiers were doing with them." Upon his return from the army, he asked a friend for a job as a carpenter. He worked for this man for several years until asked to go to the city to build houses. He thought this was too far away and didn't like big cities, so he quit and got another job in his home area. At the time of his marriage in 1951 he was working for a coal yard but lost his job the week after he was married. After a few weeks of hunting, he went back to working for the original carpenter and has worked for him for the past fifteen years in his home town.

Mr. M. says he met his wife in a movie theater one evening. When asked what attracted him to marry her he said, "That is a very hard question, I don't know." He says that now he appreciates her because she is a good cook and takes good care of the children. He courted his wife by taking her to the movies, going to visit the neighbors, driving in the countryside, and going to ball games. He can remember proposing to her while driving one Sunday but cannot remember anything that he said or she said. They had no plans for the number or sex of children which they wanted prior to marriage. He says their sexual adjustment was satisfactory and that now intercourse once a week is enough for him although during the earlier years of their marriage he was "more of a man." He was willing to have "as many children as the good Lord would give" but also feels it is about time to stop now.

It is the impression of the interviewer that Mr. M. is a plain simple man. His ego strength seems to be adequate to meet the needs of his situation, limited as it is, though he admits that he cannot stand the stresses of the larger world around him and goes to pieces when he comes into the city and gets lost in traffic. His affect was appropriate. He seemed somewhat uncomfortable with the examiner, though he was cooperative and able to respond. In the joint interview of a family he seemed to offer little support to his wife in her explanation of her emotional problems. He does take an active part in the affairs of the home, playing ball and other games with the children and disciplining them when he is there. He takes the family to church nearly every Sunday and is happy that the children are showing interest in it. His insight into Jeff's and the family's problems is quite limited, though he realizes that the main problem of not wanting to go to school is related to his wife and her grief over her mother's death. One recent sign of awareness of his wife's need for support is the fact he gave her a box of candy at Valentine's Day this year, which was a complete surprise to her and made her very happy.

Mental Status Examination:

Jeff was neatly dressed in a blue suit, in contrast to the plain clothing of his parents. He appeared sad and stood clinging to his mother in the waiting room. When it was suggested that he come along to play, he became sullen with downcast eyes and said, "I won't go." His mother was invited to the examining room with us. Jeff immediately showed interest in the toys but then refused to play and sat with arms folded on a chair. When it was suggested that the mother leave the room, he suggested the alternative of playing with the toys in the hall where his mother was taking her MMPI test. On the second visit he readily and happily accepted leaving his mother to go and play. While in the room, he said several times, "That other room didn't have as many toys in it as this one" and "The reason children don't like to play so well the first time is because they don't know how much fun it is at the clinic."

Jeff's orientation and perception are good. Neuromuscular integration is normal. Thought processes are orderly and he verbalizes well. Intelligence seems to be average. His fantasy play and other comments show a preoccupation with people being hurt or killed, especially the mother. He spontaneously began drawing a brown figure in the shape of a house which he said was a mountain with rocks falling off it, crushing the cars below and hurting the people. He also commented that the doll house looked like a tornado had hit it. He said it was dangerous to live on the edge of the table as the people in the doll house did because they might be hit by a tornado. He was frequently distracted by the sound of sirens, saying that the ambulance was going to pick up sick people who had been hurt in an accident, or there were fire trucks, or that they might be going to pick up sick people or going to an accident. He said they saw a wreck on the way home in which someone was killed, and his mother had seen a car rolled over on the way today. While playing with the truck, moving the furniture out of the doll house, he put a baby in the house, saying that it might get hit by the truck. He went on to say that the mother might also be hit by the truck and die. Then the family would have no mother.

He fired the gun and said he wished he could have one but that his mother wouldn't let him have any because she was afraid of guns. He drew a picture of a boat, and though he could not see the people on it he made up a story about a family there. He said the people were happy on the boat, but some might be sad because they couldn't get up on top and pilot the boat for fear of being thrown off and drowned. This would make the family sad and they would "kick other people" and then cry. He expressed the thought that if the baby were kicked he might die or if the husband were kicked that he might kick back at the mother. He said that the boy might help his mother if she were sad by staying home or by buying presents for her instead of going outside and playing.

He said his favorite television show was "Casper the Ghost." He said that Casper had no friends and was always trying to make friends but whenever they found out he was a ghost they would be scared away. He also related a TV story about a rocket ship which crashed and resulted in injury for the occupants. His three wishes were for material things: to have a gun like the one in the playroom, to have a car of his own, and to have another car, a pick-up truck. He asked me to copy a picture of a bear from a book, and as I was doing it he said "Make it sad" although the bear in the book had a smile. When asked why the bear was sad, he said, "Mommy won't let him have a gun." When drawing a person he drew a vague figure and first said it was a mom and later said it was a little girl who was in a bear costume for Halloween.

Jeff appears to be struggling with the fear that he will not grow up to be a man. His desire to break away from the mother's dominance is shown by his interest in masculine playthings and in his ability to leave her happily at the second visit. His fear of separation would appear to be largely a reaction formation against hostility aroused by conflict with the mother. However, his grandmother's death and the mother's current depression give his fear of her injury or death some reality basis. His comments about guns and the bear suggest that, at a more unconscious level, conflicts over Oedipal wishes and castration anxiety contribute to his discomfort.

Diagnostic Conference

Formulation:

Jeff's symptoms are separation anxiety. The mother appears to have been a rather self-effacing woman all her life, dependent for approval on the maternal grandmother, in particular, but less favored than her sickly younger sister. She has shown symptoms of depression at least since Jeff's birth, compounded recently by the death of MGM. She would appear to regard Jeff ambivalently as the child who was hard to bear and ended her childbearing capability yet as the person from whom she must receive support and approval now that MGM is gone. The mother holds him close and is afraid to let him go. The father is a rather inadequate, dependent person, able to function only in his unchanging, simple home community, and incapable of giving his wife the amount of support and approval she needs. Jeff appears to be ready to break away from his mother's dominance. The mother seems to desire help with her feelings of inadequacy and dependency and should be able to benefit from therapy. The father shows little interest in help for himself but may possibly be encouraged to support the mother a little more than he has in the past.

Conference Recommendations:

1. Jeff is very ready for active play sessions which would involve handling his feelings concerning aggression and dependency. He particularly needs to express and better understand his relationship with his mother, whom he sees as not allowing him to be an adequate male.

2. Mrs. M. should be seen in therapy by a therapist who might offer her support, initially recognize the frustration of her dependency needs, and gradually help her to turn to her husband and perhaps those outside her home for such satisfaction. It is difficult to determine at this point how much insight this woman may gain into her depression.

3. The father should be seen only occasionally and then probably with his wife and her therapist in an effort to help him be more giving and supportive of the wife.

4. Jeff should return to school immediately. The principal should be contacted and urged to allow the child to attend school even though he may not be able to pass the first grade. He should then stay the entire school day and, if he becomes upset, be allowed to go to the principal's office until he regains control and

once again can return to the classroom. The child should come to the disposition conference and be reassured that he can go to school and that his mother will be there when he gets home.

(Signed) Conference Chairman

Disposition Conference with Parents:

Mr. and Mrs. M. were approximately one hour late because of Mr. M's fear of driving in the city. The mother accepted very easily the idea that she was depressed and it was her need to have the child home which was precipitating and intensifying the boy's school phobia. She accepted individual treatment for herself. Jeff has returned to school. Again, it seems quite apparent that the mother's concerns are most important in this area. She was very worried about how much he will cry at school. The father was supported in his desire to have the child help him do carpentry work around the house, such as building a dog house for a new stray dog Jeff had found. Treatment hour at 1:00 P.M. or morning would be best for the family.

Treatment Conference
(Three Months after the Diagnostic Conference)

Current Working Formulation and Progress:

Child: Jeff has been seen for twelve hours during the past three months. Initially he was tense and shaky. He tried to get me involved in games with him such as pool but was so tense that he couldn't play. For instance, at pool he couldn't hold the cue steady enough to shoot. I discouraged him from the game and gave him more physical distance. The overt anxiety cleared after several sessions. He then became demanding, seeking gifts and gratifications. He wanted to take various toys home. He always wanted to go to another office to find a different toy from what was present in my office. When restricted to my office and the toys therein, he accepted the restriction and now is less demanding. He plays with the burp guns and dart guns, shooting at the targets on the door. He plays with the building blocks, trucks, softball, and bat. He usually plays by himself and verbalizes happenings at home and things that he has seen and done. At some time during the therapy hours he gets me involved in his games.

Each time there has been a siren outside, Jeff would comment, "There goes another ambulance." When I asked him more about this he would change the subject quickly, until recently he said he saw an ambulance on the road with someone inside it. He then said it made him think of his grandmother, who died in November. He said that the doctor hadn't gotten there in time to save his grandmother. Each time he heard the ambulance he thought of that and hoped the doctor would get there to save whoever was hurt. He didn't know why the doctor hadn't gotten there to save his grandmother, but the doctor was a slowpoke. He denied anger about the doctor. Several therapy hours later, when Jeff commented on a siren he heard, I asked him if he was feeling bad when he heard the sirens. He replied, "I don't get that feeling anymore, I just say phooey on grandma. She's dead. What's the use of thinking about her? She can't come back to life. I don't even dream about her anymore. Besides, who would want to go through one of those spells again. You know, that spell about grandma."

Jeff has always avoided talking about his mother and any worries he may have about her or the rest of the family. He discussed having to take the first grade over and seems to have accepted it. He said he didn't fail and he didn't pass. They just wanted him to take it over because he missed so much school. He says he doesn't care because he will learn more anyway.

The report from school indicates regular attendance and improvement in his relations with both peers and adults. His attention span and attitude toward his studies are improving. However, he will be retained in the first grade because he has missed too much to make up the work.

In summary, I think Jeff has made some progress, at least in therapy hours. He is less overtly anxious, more independent, and has ventilated a lot of feelings. Although he uses denial extensively, he verbalizes some insight.

Mother: She is without reservation in coming for help for herself and recognizes that there is a connection between her problems and Jeff's problems. Initially she expressed much emotion in the hours, talking about her anger at the demands people make upon her, especially a very disturbed, neglected neighbor child. After this was somewhat resolved, there was a plateau for a few weeks in April and May. When we began talking about her treatment of Jeff as a special child, this opened the subject of her relationship to MGM and the dam broke. For a number of weeks we have discussed her feelings of loss since MGM's death. She has worked through a great many feelings and is very busily involved in church and family activities. She is a very simple, rural woman who seems to have low average intelligence, is not superstitious, but tends to use somewhat illogical cause-and-effect reasoning. She has agreed that she should come for treatment even if Jeff discontinues his treatment. She is aware of a great deal of improvement in both the boy and herself.

Conference Recommendations:

Jeff is symptom-free at this time. The boy has quite satisfactorily worked through his feelings about his grandmother's death. While he is unable to talk in therapy about his mother, he no longer clings to her or her to him. It might be necessary to explore more fully his relations with his parents. However, in view of his current freedom from anxiety and the fact his therapist is leaving the clinic, we will discontinue therapy for the time being.

Mrs. M. is currently discussing her relationship with her mother and is progressing satisfactorily. She should continue at least a few more sessions until she has better insight into her feelings about her mother.

(Signed) Conference Chairman

Final Treatment Conference
(Approximately six months after the beginning of therapy)

Since the last treatment review, Mrs. M. has been seen for an additional eleven sessions at weekly intervals and one final session after a lapse of six weeks. She discussed her earlier relationships with her mother and her current feelings about her siblings. She has become quite direct, at times, almost impulsive, in verbalizing her anger to the therapist, to her husband, and to her siblings. She has become able to hold her own in family arguments without excessive guilt, and her depression has abated. Her excessive somatization has lessened and she now follows her doctor's advice. Recent part-time employment out of the home has contributed much to her sense of well-being.

Both parents and school report Jeff to be doing well. Case closed. No further treatment needed.

(Signed) Conference Chairman

ASSAULTIVE BEHAVIOR IN A SEVEN-YEAR-OLD

Name: Granville A.

Birth Date: 12-29-59   Age: 7½ years

School: Lyman Elementary

Religion: Protestant

Referred By: Family physician, Dr. A. W.

Family		Relation to Patient	Age	Occupation or Grade
Father	Unknown			
Mother	Mary A.	Mother	29	Unemployed
Children	Granville	Patient	7½	First grade
	Ellen	Half-sister	3	
	Sybille	Half-sister	2	

Others Living in the Home:

Maternal grandmother, age 52
Stepmaternal grandfather, age 59

Presenting Problem:

Behavior problems at home and school. Until four months ago was in parochial school where he choked, pinched, and jumped on other children. Minds the teacher but not for long.

Course of Symptoms and Current Adjustment of Child:

The patient is a 7½-year-old Negro male. His mother dates the onset of present difficulty to about four months ago. Actually it was at this time that the mother realized the magnitude of the child's problem.

In March of this year, the mother received a call from the parochial school and was informed of his expulsion. The person who called indicated to the mother that the patient had been involved in numerous fights and had been observed kicking, fighting, and choking other students. It was felt by the school that the patient should be transferred to another facility.

The mother states that this all came as quite a shock to her. Although she knew her son was having some difficulty academically in school, she had no idea of the aggressive behavior of which she was told. The child was then transferred to the Lyman public school, where he was assigned a male teacher. School reports indicate that he related rather well to this individual. His grades, however, were such that he is being retained in the first grade.

Granville is the oldest of three children.

having two half-sisters, ages 3 and 2. His mother has never been married. She states that Granville has always been "a mischievous child," but she has never considered him to be bad. When the 3-year-old half-sister was born, however, Granville would attempt to push the baby off his mother's lap and take the baby's bottle. He would say on occasion, "Mama, you don't need that baby, I'm your baby." The patient in recent years seemed to have adapted quite well to his half-sisters and plays with them.

The patient's mother and half-sisters came to this area approximately two years ago at the insistence of MGM. The patient was originally enrolled at the parochial kindergarten because "they taught religion" and "they had a school bus so he wouldn't have to walk." Apparently he was believed to be ready for first grade, having had no difficulty in kindergarten.

The mother describes the patient as having a hot temper. He gets angry quite easily whenever things don't go his way. Frequently, he will cry when frustrated. He can offer no reasons to her about his difficulties with other children. Also the mother indicates that the patient, who was toilet trained by two years of age, has been enuretic at a frequency of every other night for the past six or seven months.

Background Information

Family Picture:

The family is currently composed of Granville, his mother Mary, and two half-sisters, all of whom reside with the maternal grandmother and the maternal step-grandfather. The patient's maternal uncle also lives with his family in the same town. There are several male cousins to whom Granville is rather close. Step-grandfather is a laborer. Mother receives welfare assistance for her children.

Preschool Developmental History:

Delivery was at home and was apparently uncomplicated. The patient had the usual childhood diseases but has had no serious illnesses requiring hospitalization. He sat at 3 to 4 months of age, walked at 11 months. He was toilet trained by 2 years of age. He has been enuretic for the past six months. He also talks a great deal in his sleep and has for some time.

School History:

(See Course of Symptoms.) School Report: "Much better behavior since transfer to public school and a male teacher. Although attendance good, he was absent the days achievement tests were given. However, in spite of improved conduct he has not grasped the basic academic skills and will be retained in the first grade. Mother seems distant and disinterested."

Medical History:

There are no significant medical illnesses in the patient's past history.

Mother:

Mary A. is a 29-year-old Negro female. She has an obvious physical deformity, a severe right scoliosis with elevation of the right scapula, making her quite short and giving her a humpbacked appearance.

Miss A. was the third of five children. She was born June 22, 1937. She has brothers four and two years older, and two and four years younger. The family originally lived in the South, and the patient's mother started school there. When she was 6 or 7 years of age, the maternal grandfather ran off with another woman. Maternal grandmother moved with her family to another state after that. Miss A., who had completed two years of grade school, was put back and had to start all over again. Apparently she had no difficulty in school until approximately 11 years of age. At that time she fell from a tree and "my spine started growing crooked." At about 13 years of age doctors put her into a brace. After that (the mother cannot remember exactly when) she was taken to Memphis, Tennessee, where she underwent surgery, following which she wore a body cast for about six months. She describes how tall she was and how good she felt when in the body cast. However, when the cast was removed, the scoliotic condition was unchanged and even worsened. During this period Miss A. became disgusted with everything and wanted to quit school. However, at her mother's insistence, she continued high school and graduated at age 19.

Miss A. enrolled in a state university but remained for only one year. She states she couldn't make it academically. She then enrolled in a trade school. While still enrolled in school, she became pregnant with the patient. She states that the father promised to marry her but he didn't. She became quite disgusted and eventually quit school. The patient was born in December, 1959. Miss A. states that prior to the pregnancy she knew very little of sex, having learned everything she knew from other girls. Her mother used to talk to her prior to that only in terms of staying away from men. The mother tried various types of pills in order to get her menstrual period started but made no active attempt to abort herself when pregnant with Granville. She states that she definitely did not want the pregnancy but accepted it. She went to live with her oldest paternal uncle and his wife and continued living there after the birth of the patient. She would share babysitting chores with the uncle's wife and was able at times to get out of the house. When Granville was five years of age, his mother became pregnant by another man. She states that she loved this man and thought that he would marry her. She has had two children by this man but no marriage. Approximately two and a half years ago, the mother was asked by the maternal grandmother to come live here. MGM had remarried when the mother was approximately 15 years of age. MGM has given her "hell" for having three illegitimate children and for failing her (MGM). Miss A. states that this used to upset her and make her quite angry but that now she simply ignores MGM.

MGM is described as a "good lady. She raised all five of us without a daddy." However, MGM continues to dominate the home. Maternal stepgrandfather is described as a good, quiet man "who has tried to help me as much as he can."

Mother started training in a vocational rehabilitation program about two weeks ago. She states that at first she didn't think she would be able to make it and this upset her a great deal. However, now she feels she can make it.

She related in a rather distant manner, showing little evidence of anxiety or concern. There is a great deal of psychomotor retardation, but she denies being depressed. On direct questioning she states she feels the fact that Granville is a Negro may have had something to do with the trouble he had in school. She indicates that other children in that school system who are Negro have complained of being intimidated by white youths.

Father:

All information about the father was obtained from the mother. She states that Granville's father now lives in the South. She feels that Granville knows who his father is because, while they lived near him, the father would sometimes stop Granville on the street and give him money. She has never talked to the patient about his father, although he has asked frequently. The mother's only description of the father is that he was a drinking man who apparently had some difficulty learning in school.

Mental Status Examination:

Granville was examined on three occasions. He was initially seen with his mother in a joint interview. He was also observed by me on several occasions while he was in the lobby in the child guidance clinic, as well as being seen for two individual playroom sessions at weekly intervals.

On each occasion, Granville was quite neat

in appearance. He rapidly scanned his surroundings in most instances. He appeared to be a bright youngster with a great deal of curiosity. Especially noteworthy was the ease with which he was able to leave his mother. In fact he often was completely oblivious to her presence. At the time of the initial interview, he shook hands with the examiner. He sat in a chair only a short time before he was up inspecting my office. He immediately picked up a dart gun and loaded it. He then called, "Mother!" When she turned around, he pointed the gun at her but did not shoot.

Granville was well oriented for the most part. However, at the initial interview, he said he was told he was going to an eye doctor. When informed of who I was, he simply nodded but offered no comment. Granville said that he was going to be retained in the first grade because he was bad, yet he could offer no source of this information. Throughout each interview, he continually shot darts either at the target on the door or at dominoes which he had lined up on the bookshelf. He would answer questions often with his back to the examiner.

He is well coordinated. His speech is usually coherent, although at times it is difficult to hear. He described a recurrent nightmare in which a black humpbacked man was going to kill him. His drawings of a man and woman were rather bizarre, with little attention paid to body form and appendages. His drawing of a woman, in fact, was quite poor. He wishes that (1) he could have a horse so that he could ride around the country, (2) he could have a cowboy suit and be a western boy so that he could shoot with a real gun, and (3) he could have a real gun so that he could show it to people and shoot it up in the sky. "I'm a good shot. Got to be a good shot by chunkin' rocks." When questioned about his mother, he would only say, "Ain't got nothing to say about her. She comes out and plays with me sometimes." He immediately began talking about guns again after this interchange. He volunteered he sleeps in the lower bunk with his mother because he fears falling out of the top bunk. He would not talk about his sisters. When he was finished playing, he would leave toys and darts on the floor. However, when reminded of this, he would immediately pick these up. It is my feeling that he will respond when limits are set, but this has probably not been done consistently in the past.

Granville feels that he must have been bad because he is being retained in the first grade. Yet in his fantasy he would like to be one of the good guys. He talks about being a sheriff or a policeman and chasing bad boys.

In summary, this 7½-year-old Negro male is quite neat in appearance. He seems preoccupied with thoughts of aggressiveness and constantly acts these out. He also seems to be preoccupied with the idea of his own badness. He appears to be of average intelligence. There appears to be a great deal of difficulty with self-identity. Also there are indications of a poor concept of women as exemplified by his mother, with whom he is quite angry.

Psychological Testing:

Tests Administered:
  Draw-A-Person Test

Wechsler Intelligence Scale for Children
Rorschach
Thematic Apperception Test
Structured Doll Play Technique

Granville is a nice-looking 7½-year-old Negro boy who was tested at the request of Dr. L. Consultation was requested primarily concerning the following questions: (1) intellectual level, (2) ability to handle aggressive impulses, (3) awareness of own difficulties, and (4) ability to work in therapy with a male therapist. Granville was cooperative although somewhat slow during the testing session, and he seemed to relate rather well to this examiner.

The predominant impression from the test material is that Granville is involved in a rather difficult and confusing relationship with his mother. He feels that to please her he must be strong and responsible or his mother will reject and/or leave him. He also feels pressured from his mother to meet some of her needs. Granville finds it quite difficult to satisfy his mother, and he feels inadequate to meet her expectations. His feelings of inadequacy are also contributed to by his perception of adult males as ineffectual and distant; he has apparently been unable to identify with an adequate male figure.

Although he tries to satisfy his mother by being a little man, at times his dependency needs become quite strong, and he feels that his mother does not try to meet them. Although feeling attached to her (perhaps neurotically so), he is quite angry at the emotional distance perceived between himself and her. As long as he is the little man, he and his mother have an adequate relationship, but when he demands dependency-need gratification, he also fears rejection. Hence, he is reluctant to express his anger about his ungratified dependency needs directly toward his mother and vents his hostility on others. For example, he is probably quite hostile toward other children. In addition, his feelings of inadequacy have been exacerbated by his experiences in school, where he feels he is rejected and scorned. The only controls over the expression of his hostility which were prominent in test data are denial and suppression, and these became inadequate rather readily; hence, aggressive outbursts are probably easily elicited from him.

With the many burdens and frustrations which Granville perceives in real life, he finds some gratification in active fantasy. Although some slightly autistic fantasy was manifested in his Rorschach responses, this was not sufficiently bizarre to suggest psychosis. He does appear to be at least moderately emotionally disturbed, with his difficulties being primarily of a neurotic and characterological nature. The amount, availability, and poor control of his hostility indicate that psychotherapy is necessary for him at this time. He appears to be a bright, sensitive boy, in spite of his history of poor school performance. Although he achieved an IQ score of only 91 on the Wechsler Intelligence Scale for Children, his talent for reasoning and sizing up situations seems indicative of above-average intellectual capacity. In addition, Granville does appear to feel discomfort about himself and his situation. Thus he appears to have talents and motivation which would be positive assets in psychotherapy.

Diagnostic Formulation:

This 7½-year-old Negro male was referred to this clinic for evaluation because of outbursts of aggressive behavior directed toward peers and because of difficulty in school. He is the oldest of three illegitimate children of his unwed mother. The patient's mother has a severe physical deformity and some disability. Granville was an unwanted child, but following his birth his mother devoted her entire attention to him. However, the mother has remained chronically unhappy, and it appears that she is constantly unable to satisfy the boy's needs. The mother became pregnant again five years after his birth. His reaction to this was one of extreme hostility which he has been unable to control adequately. His behavior at school represents an expression of hostility. Also, because of cultural variables, this child was not prepared for entrance into the school situation. The lack of a father figure is confusing to him and has given him no one with whom to identify. The mother clinically appears detached, distant, and somewhat suspicious of the motives of others. Granville's problems at this time represent a behavior disorder which assumes the pattern of a characterological disorder. However, fixed patterns do not seem well established yet. The mother's personal and social problems and the current living situation are continuous stimulants of his aggressive behavior and deprive him of controls and identification models.

Treatment Recommendations:

1. Granville is an attractive Negro boy with many social and cultural strikes against him. He needs an adequate masculine figure with whom to identify. He seems to be seeking ways to express himself more appropriately and be accepted. He will be seen weekly by a male therapist. In addition we will explore the resources in his community for group recreation experiences outside the home.

2. Miss A. should have an evaluation of her physical deformity. In view of the many advances in orthopedic surgery in the past twenty years, a current evaluation is needed. Miss A. will also be seen weekly at this clinic. She will no doubt resist exploration of her feelings and personal relationships. Help will be offered with her medical and vocational problems and in matters of the home management of Granville. If a trusting relationship can be established, it may be possible to explore her problems with her mother and with men.

Disposition Conference:

Miss A. was seen and the staff recommendations were reviewed with her. She readily accepted the idea of weekly therapy sessions for Granville. She was a bit more reluctant about sessions for herself but agreed to come. She accepted an appointment for evaluation by the

orthopedic department. First therapy session
scheduled for 2:00 P.M. on August 20.*

SCHOOL FAILURE OF AN EIGHT-YEAR-OLD

Name: Jimmy D.

Birth Date 8-2-58   Age: 8 years

School: Escalante Elementary

Religion: Protestant

Referred By: Dr. L., the mother's psychiatrist

Family		Relation	Age	Occupation
Father	Harold D.	Father	28	Laborer
Mother	Sylvia D.	Mother	28	Secretary
Children	Jimmy D.	Patient	8	Second grade
	No siblings			

---

* In therapy, Granville rather quickly formed a very positive attachment to his therapist. In play-acting he reviewed many of his conflicts about his mother and himself. School behavior improved both socially and academically. However, at home he continued to be caught in the conflicts of the mother and grandmother.

It required intensive casework to help Miss A. overcome her extreme pessimism and accept rather extensive and prolonged orthopedic treatment. Upon learning that Miss A. would require extended bed care, a conference was arranged with her, the grandmother, the local public health nurse and the welfare department to plan for her convalescence and the continued care of the children. Arrangements were made for Granville to be placed in a group home where he could continue receiving psychotherapy. The grandmother agreed to continue to provide a home for the mother and sisters with assistance from the public health nursing service.

At our last contact Miss A. was ambulatory in a brace, had had some training at Goodwill Industries and was looking for part-time employment near her home. Granville's adjustment in the group home had many ups and downs, ranging from good to marginal at times. It is not anticipated that he will return to live with his mother until he has achieved considerably more maturation and stability. It is possible that he may have to continue living in the group home indefinitely if his mother is unable eventually to provide a home for herself and her children independent of her own mother.

Presenting Problem:

Problem with school — i.e., failing courses.

Course of Symptoms and Current Adjustment of Child:

The parents state that Jimmy has had to repeat the first grade of school, did poorly during his repeat year, and is now doing very poorly in the second grade. Mrs. D. discussed her concern about Jimmy's school problem with her psychiatrist, who referred the family to this clinic.

Jimmy began first grade at age 6 and did poorly from the beginning. He brought home papers with poor grades but was not involved in any disciplinary problems or absenteeism. The mother states that she was not overly concerned at the time because she felt that perhaps Jimmy was still a little bit too young to accept the full responsibilities for achieving in school. He failed virtually every course and after repeating the first grade was promoted to the second grade because of "social pressure" and because the teacher "wanted to get rid of him." With further questioning, the parents also reported Jimmy has problems relating with other children. He is unable to form close or lasting friendships because he imposes overly strong demands on his friends in play activity, and when they do not abide by his demands he becomes violently angry with them.

Both the mother and father feel that a poor family environment and two episodes of acute psychotic reactions in the mother have contributed most significantly to Jimmy's problems. The father is, however, considerably more outspoken about this. Both parents express guilt feelings and now want to repay him for all the "lack of love" which he experienced during the more turbulent periods of their relationship. They do this primarily by not imposing disciplinary limits on the child. When he does transgress the few behavioral limits they have for him, they do not punish him. The father states that during the first episode of acute psychosis that the mother suffered, she attempted to handle the school problem by "beating Jimmy." Father states that she would beat him so viciously with a belt that he would bleed from the wounds on his back. This did not continue very long, as the father would not allow it. Jimmy developed an overt fear of his mother which persists to the present. The father states the child would often beg not to be left alone with the mother, as he was afraid of what she would do to him. The more recent attempts by the parents to handle this school problem have been primarily by helping with schoolwork. This, however, has not proved successful.

The parents still argue about discipline. The father feels that Jimmy should have more rigid behavioral limitations than he does but that he should not be punished physically for misbehavior. The mother, on the other hand, feels that Jimmy should not be limited by rigid behavioral controls, but when he does misbehave she spanks him very severely with a belt. The parents observed Jimmy playing with his genitals about one year ago. This behavior continued, and the father admonished him not to do it. The mother's approach to this was one of "educating him," and she states that she explained to Jimmy the physiology of reproduction. Jimmy has been sleeping with his mother

during the past year while father has been working the night shift. According to the father,
Jimmy says that his mother makes him sleep with
her.

Background Information

Family Picture:

The father is currently employed as a laborer
and has an income of $109.00 per week. The mother
is employed as a secretary at a small store and
has a take-home pay of $58.00 per week. The fam-
ily lives in a five-room rented home which has
two bedrooms. The family does not share in any
activity together. There appears to be no interaction between the mother and father or between
the mother and Jimmy. The significant interaction which does occur in this family appears to
be limited to the relationship between Jimmy
and his father.

Preschool Developmental History:

Mrs. D. became pregnant about one year after
the marriage, and both parents state that although the pregnancy was not planned they were
desirous of having a child in the near future
and therefore the fact of the pregnancy was well
accepted. The pregnancy and delivery were uneventful. Jimmy's birth weight was 8 pounds, 6
ounces, and the immediate postnatal course was
uneventful. There were no birth defects or difficulties with eating or development. Jimmy
sat up at about 6 months, talked at 9 months,
walked at 16 months, and was toilet trained at
about 2 years.

School Report:

"Jimmy daydreams and plays instead of doing

his work. Repeated first grade. Now in second-grade placement, but achievement is near failure. California Mental Maturity Test last year rated IQ level as average. Recent Stanford Primary Achievement, Form W, results were: Reading 1.9, Spelling 2.0, and Arithmetic 1.4. Child overactive and distractable."

Medical History:

No serious illnesses or injuries.

Mother:

Mrs. D. is a slightly obese female who appears her stated age of 28. Her affect fluctuated appropriately with the mood of discussion, but she did not exhibit the normal full range of variation. Her face was almost masklike at times, and she stared blankly on many occasions.

Her general attitude is one of sincere desire to elucidate the dynamics of the problem and if possible to determine methods of improving the situation. Her perception and orientation were normal, and there were no detectable disturbances of reality testing. There were no evidences of bizarre thought processes. However, the session was quite structured in the sense that the interviewer posed specific questions.

The MGM is 66 and the MGF is 72; both living and well. There are seven children in the family including Mrs. D. Her brother, 35 years old, is the one who now manages the D. family's financial problems and played an active role in having her hospitalized on both occasions. Mrs. D's interaction with the remainder of her siblings is apparently not significant. The mother describes the MGM as kind, loving, and an ideal housewife and mother. The MGM sees Jimmy approximately once a week and apparently has an amiable relationship with him. The MGF is described as intelligent, strong, domineering, and a leader. Mrs. D. states that she was the MGF's favorite child because she appeared to be the most intelligent of the children. MGF is a retired minister. Mrs. D. was an honor student and socially active in high school. She planned to attend college but is vague about why she didn't. The mother experienced her menarche at the age of 12 years. She was never really taught anything about the physiology of sex at home. She did have dates in high school and appeared to be quite popular. After dating her husband for about five months, they indulged in sexual intercourse and this was the mother's first sexual experience. She states that her sexual relationships at that time were not satisfactory and have never become so, in that she has never experienced an orgasm. When asked what she liked about the patient's father, she states she was attracted to him physically in "an air force uniform."

According to both parents, the marriage began with a stormy course. The father admittedly had an inferiority complex, and this manifested itself as lack of desire to dominate or manage the home situation and lack of desire to socialize outside of the family. The mother states that because of "incompatibility regarding personality" the marriage began with difficulties. The father's introvert personality and inferiority complex persisted in spite of her attempts to get him to socialize more actively and to develop a higher self concept. The mother worked during most of the marriage, including the month before and shortly after Jimmy's birth. Although they openly discussed divorce, they merely continued in their relationship of virtual isolation from one another. Jimmy was cared for by a babysitter during this time. The mother volunteers that she became totally involved in her work and church activities because she "didn't want to go home to the husband I hated." Although this entire period of life is rather vague to the mother now, she states that in June of 1962 she felt that she could not live with her husband any longer. She took her son and traveled south to a school for missionaries. She intended to enroll in the school and travel to some foreign country as a missionary. After five days, she called her local minister, who reported her location to the family and started the proceedings for the mother's first commitment to a mental hospital. She received "intensive psychotherapy and electroshock therapy" for three months. Apparently the mother remained relatively stable until November, 1965, when Jimmy was 6½ years old. This was the time in which Mrs. D. violently whipped Jimmy with a belt. During this period she had extramarital relationships on numerous occasions with different men in the community. The father is not aware of this. After a period of approximately six months of acting out and the development of manifest symptoms such as distortion of reality testing, Mrs. D. was again hospitalized for six weeks. She states that prior to her recent hospitalization, sex was the most important thing in her married life. Now, however, she feels companionship and social interaction are equally significant. She submits herself to her husband purely as a tool for releasing his sexual drives and overtly ridicules him during his period of excitement shortly before his orgasm. Prior to the mother's most recent acute psychotic episode, she was the manager of financial affairs in the family. At the time of hospitalization her brother took over the management of finances and has continued to manage the family finances to the present time.

There has been virtually no interaction between the father and mother or between the mother and Jimmy during the past year. The father has been working the night shift, the mother has been working days, and they see each other during waking hours only about 45 minutes to one hour each day. The mother consistently goes to bed about seven o'clock in the evening, and when the father is at home he and Jimmy sit up alone and watch television. The mother works on Saturday and sleeps most of Sunday.

The mother states that she feels much of Jimmy's problems are probably manifestations of his disordered family life, and she feels that her two episodes of psychosis and the periods leading up to her hospitalization probably played significant and detrimental roles in his psychological development. She wants Jimmy to graduate from high school and get a college education. She would like the clinic to elucidate some of the problems contributing to Jimmy's current difficulties and if possible give her methods for improving. She is willing to alter her behavior and play an active role to the degree of coming to the clinic regularly, perhaps once a week, if this is what the clinic recommends.

Father:

The father is a well-developed, slightly obese male who appears his stated age of 28. He related fairly well with the interviewer. However, there was very poor eye contact. He looked at the floor while he was speaking and displayed mild anxiety when asked direct questions. His verbalizations, on the other hand, were surprisingly lucid. He feels that the problem is directly related to the psychosis of the mother. He has a sincere desire for advice and is willing to modify his behavior, if necessary, to improve the situation.

The PGF is a 55-year-old laborer. He is a chronic alcoholic who was vicious during his drunken stupors and often beat the children and the PGM. The PGPs divorced when the father was 6 years old, and he went to live with his grandparents. During drunken episodes the PGF made fun of the father and of the other children in the areas of personal work and achievement. The father always did poorly in school and did not receive encouragement from the PGF but rather humiliation. This type of repeated negative stimulus nurtured a feeling of inferiority and helped to develop his introverted type of personality. There is very little current interaction between the PGF and the father and no significant contact between the PGF and Jimmy.

The PGM is 52 years old, living and well, and is described by the father as loving, warm, and intelligent. The PGM has successfully entered many writing contests and apparently has been employed as a writer. Although the father claimed affection for his mother, he never was able to confide his personal problems to either of his parents. The father is the oldest of four siblings. He states his sister and one brother have escaped the humiliation imposed by the PGF and have developed an extrovert type of personality. However, the 16-year-old brother is described by the father as being very much like himself, only worse. This brother is extremely shy and avoids social interaction at all costs.

The father always disliked school and did poorly but completed high school. Within the past year or two he has begun to feel he has a greater potential than indicated by his achievements. Therefore, he is learning a new trade as a mold designer. He was engaged to one girl about one year before meeting his wife. This engagement did not continue because the girl moved out of state. He had his first sexual experience with his wife about one month prior to their marriage and has never had any sexual experiences with other women. The father has been very tolerant of the mother's domineering and often abusive attitude toward himself and Jimmy. Recently he has begun to feel his intelligence to be equal to his wife's. This has led to more open clashes with his wife, regarding decisions in family affairs. Except for occasional sexual contact, the father and mother seldom talk or associate with each other.

In 1962 the father suffered a "mild nervous breakdown" manifested by anxiousness and depression. He was treated by a private physician with Stelazine for about six months and feels he recovered. He attributes most of Jimmy's problems to the stormy home environment provided by the mother. If he and the mother are divorced he would like to have Jimmy. He has discussed this with the boy, who said he would like to live with his father. Mr. D. desires a diagnosis and counseling from the clinic. He is willing to modify his behavior and be seen in the clinic regularly for some period of time if we so advise. He seems rather pessimistic about the future of his marriage.

Mental Status Examination:

Jimmy D. is an 8-year-old boy. He has small features, a crew cut, and wears rather thick glasses. He is appropriately dressed in cotton school clothes. He is well oriented. Neuromuscular integration and coordination are good, but there was moderate disturbance in right-left orientation under pressure. He is able to catch and throw a ball vigorously.

Jimmy initially related to the examiner in a teasing manner. He would sit in his chair and smile, giggling occasionally, and would not initiate any spontaneous activity. Later in his play he became active and animated while shooting a dart gun at the blackboard. He fired it at a circular target and at a "monster."

Jimmy told me that he had come to the clinic because he didn't have any friends at school and that most of his play in his neighborhood is with four neighborhood boys: Eddie, age 7; Allen, age 10; Robbie, age 6; and Jerry, age 11. He said of the four that he liked Allen, the 10-year-old, best because he and Allen like to play astronaut and climb trees, playing like they are in space ships. He said that he did not like Robbie, the 6-year-old, because he is too little and "can't talk right."

Jimmy's fantasy life concerned monsters, being eaten up by monsters, being taken away at night by a burglar, being taken to the burglar's house and then killed, being burned to death, and falling in a sewer. He tells of a "funny dream" wherein he dreamed that he fell into a sewer while trying to get a ball. While in the sewer, he told his friend Robbie to go get—at this point he made a slip and said "my mother," quickly changing it to "my father." "He came and called the police. They came and got me out. We went into the house and watched TV and then I went to sleep. Then I woke up and dreamed that I saw penguins walking into my room, and they laughed at me for sleeping."

In the Raven's Controlled Projection Test, Jimmy told of a 10-year-old boy, named Allen, who liked to play astronaut. Allen's mother and father got angry at him because he got in the trash cans and scattered the trash all over the yard. Allen got mad because his parents were angry. He ran away to Jimmy's house. Allen was especially mad because his parents went after him. Allen's secret was that he had a cat that he was hiding from his mom and dad because his mom and dad wouldn't let him keep it. He took his friends to the cat and they played with it. Allen used to tell stories about going up into space. He told his friends that he had been up into space. This was not true, but he wanted his friends to think so. He told his mother and father that he was sick. He was not sick, but he told them this so he would not have to go to school. Allen was very scared and frightened because the dog bit him. After Allen went to bed he thought about a monster. He was afraid that the monster would get him. When he fell asleep he dreamed that the monster did get him and that the monster ate him. He woke up because he was so frightened of the monster. Allen's three wishes were for a space capsule, a kitty-cat, and a space suit, and if Allen had a lot of money he would buy a box of toys. Allen also wanted to be a dog because a dog can bite. Jimmy said he liked the story because Allen was very much like him. They both liked astronauts. Allen was different from him because Allen ran away from home and had a kitty-cat.

Jimmy said that he had trouble making friends because they like to start fights and they don't like him because he failed the first grade. He likes to play with boys because girls like to play house. He has been sleeping with his mother most every night up until last week when his dad got a new job. At night he fears that a man, a burglar, will come and steal him and take him away and kill him. If he saw a burglar he would holler and tell his dad to get his gun.

Jimmy was afraid to come to the child guidance clinic because he feared that I would put a stick down his throat and he would choke. He said, "I worry about dying a lot. I worry that it would hurt. I wouldn't like it." He said that he first started worrying about dying when his family moved three years ago. An attic of a barbershop burned across the street from their house, and he began to worry that he might catch fire, burn up, and die. If he died he wouldn't get to see anybody anymore. He said that he

didn't like their town because it has too many
people and they are always having fires. He
wishes he could move where Grandma and Grandpa
live.

His mother and father fight about "little
things" like "if Daddy leaves a sock around,
Mommy gets mad at him. One time Mommy hit Daddy
over the head with a toy gun and broke it. Mommy
also gets mad at Daddy because Daddy won't help
her bring in the groceries." His favorite parent is his father. He enjoys taking company
trips with his father. His mother was a patient
in the hospital. "When Mommy was sick she ran
away from home with me and we went to Georgia."
I asked how his mother acts while sick and he
replied, "She gets mean, she acts mean." Jimmy
said, "I would like to have an older brother and
sister. They could play with me when I don't
have no friends. My dad plays with me. We wrestle
once in a while but not often enough. I keep
trying to get him to and he won't. He's too busy
watching TV. I like "The Green Hornet" because
they fight and stuff. Mommy likes to go to bed
every night at seven-thirty. Daddy and I watch
television together."

When asked to draw a picture, Jimmy drew first
a house, saying he could draw a house better
than anything else. He then drew a figure with
a smiling face standing in front of the house.
When I asked him to draw his family, he drew
his father to the extreme left and labeled it
Harold. Jimmy drew his mother in the center,
labeling it Sylvia, and drew himself at the
right, labeling it Jimmy. The father and Jimmy
look exactly alike except that the father is
taller and Jimmy has bigger feet. All figures
have a smiling face and all are complete.

Jimmy particularly enjoyed playing pass with me with the basketball and became very friendly toward me as we were doing this. Regarding his problems, he said he wished the other kids liked him better and that he didn't have to worry about dying. He did not think he has any serious problems with his studies or with his parents.

Psychological Testing:

PROCEDURES USED:

Wechsler Intelligence Scale for Children (partial) Bender Visual Motor Gestalt Test

Jimmy, age 8-3, was tested primarily to obtain a basic estimate of his intellectual capacity. The complete WISC was not given. Prorated IQ estimates were made based on the information, comprehension, vocabulary, picture completion, block design, and coding subtests. The results obtained yielded a verbal IQ of 103, performance IQ of 82, and a full-scale IQ of 92. The test results suggest a child who is somewhat impulsive in interpersonal relationships and often confused by the demands of academic tasks. It is the examiner's impression that a high level of anxiety and short attention are interfering with his academic achievement, but a trial of therapy or further projective testing would be necessary to confirm this impression.

Diagnostic Conference Formulation:

Jimmy is an 8-year-old male whose poor academic performance and difficulties in forming satisfactory peer relationships seem to have resulted from the chronic emotional turmoil in his home. He has experienced parental ambivalence and confusion about agression, sex, male-female roles, and child-adult relations. He may be afraid to commit himself to his schoolwork or his friends because he sees the world as very unsettled and offering no clear-cut guides. His poor attention to schoolwork is probably the result of preoccupation in fantasy with the aggression which he sees everywhere. Pretending everyone is happy, moving to the grandparents, or having siblings are all fantasied solutions for lessening his fears. In spite of many traumatic emotional experiences, Jimmy has adequate reality contact and still desires interhuman contact.

Mrs. D. has had two hospitalizations for acute psychotic reactions. She has intellectual understanding of her problems with her husband and child. However, her capacity for empathic human relations is limited. Although she functions satisfactorily in her work, her hold on reality is tenuous and she appears unable to find personal gratification in either the mother or wife role.

Mr. D. has a poor self concept and has always been an underachiever. Since his wife's illnesses became so acute he has begun to question his inferiority to her. Even so, he is afraid − or, for other reasons, is only marginally able −to cope with her aggression or to manage the financial and other affairs of family living. At present he desires to improve things but is unable to help either himself or Jimmy.

Staff Recommendations:

1. Individual psychotherapy for Jimmy. We will try to offer him male identification, an opportunity to ventilate his fears, and help in understanding his world.

2. Unless Jimmy's environment can be improved, his therapy will not be effective. It

may be necessary to place him out of the home, but first intensive counseling with the parents should be tried.

Mr. D. will be seen weekly by a therapist to help him achieve a better appraisal of his abilities, to encourage him to assume a stronger role in managing family affairs, and to help him find ways of protecting Jimmy from Mrs. D's irrational outbursts and erratic behavior.

As requested by Mrs. D's physician, we will assume the management of her drug therapy. She is not at this point a candidate for insight psychotherapy. Rather we will try to capitalize upon her intellectual ability to help her accept more decisive behavior from the father and to suppress her impulsive and aggressive behavior.*

---

*The reader will be interested to know that this family accepted the treatment recommendations of the staff. Initially, Jimmy was very frightened, jittery, and evasive in his therapy sessions. However, after a few weeks he indulged in fantasy play and direct discussion of his family and school problems. He changed from being overtly aggressive with peers to being submissive and a scapegoat. More recently, he has formed a few normal give-and-take friendships. The school reported marked improvement, and with considerable effort on his part Jimmy passed to the next grade.

The mother attends clinic regularly. She became increasingly delusional in her thinking and conversations. As a result she lost her job, but another hospitalization was averted by adjustment of her medication. She has stopped sleeping with Jimmy and leaves his discipline to the father. She remains overtly hostile to the father but moved with him to a house nearer his work and away from her relatives under his threat of leaving.

Mr. D. is progressing in his new job and doing satisfactorily in night school. He remains very shy and uncertain, seeking much advice and reassurance. At present he is uncertain whether or not to continue the marriage. He has taken the financial responsibilities from his brother-in-law and no longer discusses his marital problems with Jimmy. He accepts the responsibility for the child's discipline.

The ultimate prognosis for the family remains somewhat uncertain, but progress to date has been encouraging.

SUMMARY

The case study method has been illustrated by three cases presented in detailed summary form, following the outline given on pages 127 and 128. This outline offers a structure for recording examination data and facilitates the diagnostic and treatment formulation when single, specific etiology of symptoms cannot be identified.

The first case illustrated a child and mother's reaction to an acute emotional stress. The second boy illustrates the result of a combination of untoward sociocultural experiences and an emotionally stressful mother-child interaction pattern. In the third instance we have reviewed a boy whose school performance was considerably below his native ability because of the chronic stress of living with psychologically ill parents. However, at this point Jimmy's school symptoms cannot be considered merely "a reaction" to an untoward environment in the sense that he would begin to perform adequately if he were removed from the home or if the marital maladjustment were resolved. There is evidence of disturbances within the boy himself as manifested by his poor object relationships, his continuous concern over aggression and violence in himself and others about him, his psychic discomfort (about which he readily told the examiner), his excessive reliance on fantasy to cope with anxiety, and a concomitant lessening of actual creative or productive activities in school and in play.

Treatment of Jeffrey, the school phobia boy, was primarily aimed at relieving his conflicts over the loss of his grandmother with no direct explanation or interpretation of his neurotically close identification with his mother. Treatment of the mother's depression and her acceptance of Jeff's strivings for independence seemed to be sufficient to permit the child's resumption of normal school performance.

Granville's treatment will not be so simple, since the formation of adequate self-identity, social concepts, and impulse control may be seriously impaired. Initially, treatment will focus upon supplying some of the social deficiencies of his environment and attenuating his anger by better dependency gratification. His mother needs to be helped to find a more gratifying life before she can begin to help her son toward a socially desirable maturation.

Jimmy D., the last case example, illustrates the need for treatment of multiple members of the family at whatever level each can effectively use help. The D. family shows a situation rather frequently seen among our clinic families in that the psychologically most disturbed member is permitted to dictate the most important family decisions. Although the chronicity of the parents' difficulties makes one cautious about the ultimate prognosis, there is every hope that the untoward effect of the parents' adjustments can be minimized for Jimmy.

Chapter 9

TRANSLATING THE DIAGNOSTIC FORMULATION INTO A NOSOLOGICAL DIAGNOSIS*

In CHAPTER 6 a method of making a diagnostic formulation from which one can make a treatment plan and a prognosis was presented. The many obstacles in developing a satisfactory scientific classification system for children's psychiatric disorders were also briefly discussed. However, a classificatory system was not presented with the case material of the first edition of this book. The author is particularly indebted to Dr. I. N. Berlin's review[15] and his personal communication pointing out that learning to use classification is indeed or should be an essential part of every child psychiatrist's training.

The literature contains many proposals for classification and many critiques of these proposals. However, instruction in the everyday pragmatic application of classification is seldom presented in the literature and is probably equally neglected by most training program faculties.

Most child psychiatrists officially use DSM-II. However, the classification of GAP #62 should be taught, learned, and

---

*Before proceeding with this chapter the reader should become acquainted with the following manuals:

1. Group for the Advancement of Psychiatry (GAP) Report #62, Psychopathological Disorders of Childhood: Theoretical Considerations and a Proposed Classification, June 1966.[33]
2. American Psychiatric Association, Diagnostic and Statistical Manual of Mental Disorders (DSM-II), 1968.[8]

used. Hopefully, an up-to-date version of GAP #62 will be incorporated in DSM-III (Note: There were 14 years between DSM-I (1952) and DSM-II (1968).) Before clarifying this somewhat contradictory stance on which classification system should be used, the rationale and usefulness of classification must be considered.

WHY CLASSIFY?

Classification enhances understanding of case material and is important for treatment. Those who rationalize that classification is contraindicated because it tends to obscure individual differences are confusing classification with formulation. Formulation deals specifically with the dynamics of an emotional disturbance in a single child. Classification orders our knowledge about disorders of childhood but does not classify children. In treatment, a complete as possible understanding of the child is mandatory. Such understanding includes not only his unique individuality but also those characteristics which he shares with others. Symptom clusters, etiology, course of symptoms, severity, theoretical constructs regarding dynamics, age differences, intellectual variations and prognosis are all essential for treatment planning. These factors also should be the bases for the "ideal" classificatory system. At this time no theory of dynamics has received general support and definitive knowledge is lacking in each of the other factors listed above as bases for both scientifically planning treatment and classification. We cannot wait for the perfect answer to all questions before initiating treatment. By the same token we cannot wait for complete information before we develop common terminology and bring order to the available knowledge. No disorder can be studied unless it is identified. Hence, further knowledge about the psychological maladies of childhood will not be produced unless we identify and classify the various afflictions as we now understand them.

To briefly reiterate the above paragraph we find that learning to classify (1) is important in learning to communicate with colleagues in the clinical and research arenas; (2) is an important, albeit not the only important, preliminary to planning treatment; and (3) is essential for the advancement of scientific knowledge about the disorders of childhood. One additional pragmatic reason for learning to classify children's disorders is that failure to do so accurately may make it impossible to collect fees from third party payors. All who read this book have had or will have a claim to an insurance company disallowed. Often the refusal to pay results from the company's inability to correctly understand the diagnosis, or terminology was used which failed to convey the seriousness of the child's disability and the necessity for professional services. The insurance companies are not obligated to understand each of us and our personal jargon. It is up to us to make ourselves understood by using the terminology which is officially accepted or most commonly understood by our professional colleagues and which most simply and completely describes the condition for which the child received services.

The third party payor is a quite recent development that requires us to communicate about patients to laymen. Formerly, our clinics and hospitals merely had to list numbers of patients or clients seen in our reports to the public and private agencies that subsidized our clinical services. If official diagnostic labels were requested by grantors, we were asked only to list the numbers seen in each of several diagnostic categories and no one questioned the accuracy of each diagnosis or the appropriateness of the treatment. Third party payors both private and public are insisting upon some method of accountability. While third party payors cannot presume to make a diagnosis or dictate the treatment, they are demanding sufficient information to be able to compare your diagnosis, your selection of treatment and your charges for various types of services with the opinions and practices of your professional peers. It is in the best interests of ourselves and our patients that we develop a common terminology mutually agreeable to other professionals and readily definable for the layman.

DSM-II (1968)

We are very indebted to our many colleagues in the American Psychiatric Association Committee on Nomenclature and Statistics who for the past 30 or more years have worked to stabilize and clarify our nomenclature. Their efforts have culminated in the publication of DSM-I (1952) and DSM-II (1968). The problems of refining terminology for textbooks and other professional literature are not limited to the field of psychiatry or just to the United States, but concern all of medicine throughout the world. For decades the World Health Organization has been promoting its "International Classification of Diseases". Many countries including the United States have found the section on mental disorders in former editions of the I.C.D. quite unsatisfactory. Representatives from APA and psychiatrists from many other countries collaborated to revise the section on mental disorders in ICD-8 (approved by the World Health Assembly in 1966 for official usage beginning 1968). The DSM-II Manual is based upon ICD-8 but is not identical with it. For practical purposes in the United States DSM-II is our officially adopted nomenclature and it, along with ICD-8, represents a giant step forward in promoting international professional understanding about mental disorders. These publications (ICD-8 and DSM-II) surely do not represent the final word on classification for world medicine, psychiatry and least of all child psychiatry. They contain many compromises and defects resulting from semantic and theoretical differences as well as gaps in knowledge. Our participation in future editions of these classificatory systems should aim toward inclusion of the most updated consensus of child psychiatrists throughout the world. In the interim, we are obliged to work with the most recently accepted nomenclature. On subsequent pages the cases previously presented in this book will be used to illustrate how DSM-II can be used and to discuss the hazards and difficulties in its use.

We must admit that DSM-II does not entirely neglect child psychiatric conditions. The manual just does not go far enough in making differentiations. Schizophrenia, childhood type, is listed. However, children and adolescents are not mentioned specifically among the listings for the neuroses, organic brain syndromes, personality disorders and psychophysiologic disorders. Do the authors mean these conditions do not occur in children or that they are identical to the illnesses as they are manifested in adults? The special section "IX, Behavior Disorders of Childhood and Adolescence (308)" recognizes children are different. These childhood disorders are described as "*more* stable, internalized, and resistant to treatment than Transient Situational Disturbances but *less* so than the Psychoses, Neuroses and Personality Disorders". The definitions of words "more" and "less" are crucial but absent from the text. It is left to individual judgment to decide when a given symptom cluster should be classified as a transient situation, a disorder more or less unique to the younger age groups, or a more classical neurosis or other stable type of disturbance. The fact that many clinics permit staff to defer making a classificatory diagnosis until treatment has terminated lessens the problem here. Just as happens in all fields of medicine, it is quite possible that clinicians of equal competence may draw different conclusions from the same clinical material. A scientific classification system merely reduces the frequency of such differences and makes it possible for scientists to communicate clearly with each other most of the time.

How should the case of Jeffrey M. (p. 129) be classified using DSM-II? Jeffrey was suffering the frequently encountered symptom picture of "school phobia". From the history of the presenting complaint and the initial mental status material obtained at the first visit the preliminary differential diagnostic considerations might be:

(*a*) Adjustment reaction of childhood, 307.1 (a self-limiting reaction to the grandmother's death)

(*b*) Overanxious reaction of childhood, 308.2 (Jeff showed about half of the symptoms listed for this diagnosis.)

(*c*) Phobic neurosis, 300.2 (intense fear of a situation which the patient consciously recognizes as no real danger to himself.)

(*d*) Obsessive compulsive neurosis, 300.3 (Jeff showed persistent intrusion of unwanted thoughts.)

Subsequent examinations and the treatment clearly reduced the differential considerations to either Adjustment Reaction or Phobic Neurosis. We felt Phobic Neurosis most accurately described the condition for which Jeffrey received treatment. Others may prefer Adjustment Reaction because Jeff was reacting to an untoward event (grandmother's death and mother's ensuing depression) and had he not had treatment so soon after symptom onset he might have recovered spontaneously. Many clinicians prefer to use the least ominous sounding diagnosis for children recognizing that labels in themselves condition people's perceptions of an individual. The term Phobic Neurosis risks implying that Jeff suffered a most serious, sometimes intractable condition and in the future he may remain more psychologically vulnerable than the treatment response suggests. Some may wish to argue that Jeff was not ill at all and the true diagnosis should be "Depression of the mother". The latter type of reasoning can be likened to a refusal to make a diagnosis of pneumonia because if exposure to virulent bacteria had not occurred no symptoms or disability would be present. In reality, Jeff and his mother were both primary patients. Each received individual therapy; the mother for her depression and Jeff for his phobia.

GAP #62 (1966)

All of the diagnostic labels considered above risk conveying an erroneous impression of Jeff's disturbance unless accompanied by qualifying and clarifying phrases. Herein lies one of the advantages of using GAP #62 classification rather than DSM-II. Using GAP we would classify Jeff's illness as follows:

(4) Psychoneurotic disorder, (b) phobic type; with symptoms (III) in affective behavior, (A-2) specific fears of going to school and harm occurring to family and (A-5) manifest separation anxiety.

The GAP classification makes a concerted albeit not totally successful effort to distinguish "Healthy Responses" and "Reactive Disorders" from the more internalized and usually more refractory disturbances. The fact that Jeff unconsciously displaced his conflicted feelings about his mother onto the school situation clearly places his illness in the psychoneurotic category. "Reactive disorders . . . . are more likely to be seen in infants and preschool children because these children are less likely to have the capacity to repress affect, internalize conflict and develop a structured psychopathology." Jeff's young age (6½ yrs.) probably accounts for his limited ability to internalize the conflict. This fact enhances the prognosis but does not change the diagnosis.

The GAP manual seems a bit cumbersome to use and still mixes phenomenology and theoretical constructs to some degree. Nevertheless, it represents a useful consensus of a large number of American child psychiatrists of differing theoretical persuasions. It could become extremely valuable if it enjoys general usage. No doubt its usage will depend upon some official recognition from the APA and WHO.

Not only does GAP more clearly define "Healthy" and "Reactive" symptoms so commonly encountered in the young, but it gives careful consideration to "Developmental Deviations". Correctly assessing developmental phenomenon is a very important but most onerous chore for child psychiatrists, pediatricians and others who offer direct services to children and adolescents. In addition the GAP report leaves no doubt that the neuroses, psychoses, personality disorders, etc. do appear in children. The establishment of these diagnoses during childhood does not yet have a great deal of predictive value for the future psychological state or vulnerability during the individual's later adult life. However, the detailed descriptions of the manifestations of these disorders in the various age groups is extremely helpful to the clinician.

SPECIAL VALUE IN GAP SYMPTOM LIST

As stated above the symptom list provides a very useful standard set of words and phrases with which to qualify diagnoses. There is unavoidable overlap of the major categories and subheadings making it sometimes difficult to decide if a particular symptom should be listed under one or the other or simultaneously under two categories. Theoretical considerations and clinical judgments still compound the categorization. For example, the clinician must use his judgment in deciding whether excessive activity should be listed under motoric disturbances of bodily functions, under manic behavior within disturbances of affective behavior or under one of the subheadings of disturbances in social behavior. In spite of this difficulty, using the symptom list clearly establishes the presence or absence of specific manifestations usually associated with the diagnosis. Such information helps to convey the seriousness of the illness at the time of the initial diagnosis and in subsequent follow-up examinations.

An additional numerical severity rating of each symptom based upon the relative incapacity engendered by a particular symptom would be extremely useful in long term follow-up studies. McConville and Purohit[52] have reported a five-point, severity rating scale based upon an estimate of the environment's reaction to the symptom. At Indiana University several groups have used a six-point severity scale based upon both an estimate of the degree of disability in the child and the environment's ability or willingness to tolerate the deviant behavior. This scale was designed by Alpern[5] for use in follow-up studies. With Dr. Alpern's permission, this severity rating scale is published for the first time here.

THE ALPERN CHILD AND ADOLESCENT SYMPTOM SEVERITY RATING SCALE

The following instructions provide guidelines for a six-point scale which allows a clinical rating of the severity of children's and adolescents' symptoms. A patient may display more than one symptom in which case a rating can be accomplished for each symptom individually.

"1" RATING (not apparent)
This rating is applied when the symptom is not apparent. The category is meant to allow for process recording of a symptom, *i.e.*, provide a way of tracing the disappearance or reappearance of a symptom.

Example: A symptom of "acting out" may have been recorded at the time of the initial diagnostic evaluation but at the time of some later case review may no longer be noted by parent, therapist, or school. Such a symptom would be rated at that time as being at "1" severity.

"2" RATING (apparent but non-significant)
This rating is applied when the symptom is apparent but not significant to the patient's functioning. Specifically, a symptom which is not detrimentally affecting a patient's peer, school, or family relationship is to be scored at the "2" level of severity.

Example: A patient suffering from a facial tic which might be obvious to the professional but does not interfere with the child's peer group functioning nor is of concern to himself or his family would be best listed at "2" severity. However, if this were indicative of a generalized anxiety state which was not recorded as a separate symptom and which was significantly affecting his ability to function in the classroom situation, the "2" rating would not be appropriate.

"3" RATING (mild severity)
This rating is to be used when a particular symptom is considered to be of sufficient severity so that it is affecting the patient's functioning and/or development. However, the effect is sufficiently mild so that this symptom alone would not require psychotherapeutic intervention.

Example: A patient's hyperactivity is having its primary effect on his school functioning so that he is achieving at an average level which is somewhat below his above-average ability level. This slight educational underachievement is not of major concern to the patient or his family.

"4" RATING (moderate severity)

This rating is to be used when a particular symptom is considered to be of sufficient severity so that it is affecting the patient's functioning and/or development *and* is sufficiently handicapping so that on the basis of the severity of this symptom alone, psychotherapeutic intervention would be indicated.

Example: A patient's sexual preoccupations have led to his peer group's families terminating their children's associations with him. Here socialization has been so restricted by the sexual symptom that it tends to forbid the development of useful peer inter-relationships.

"5" RATING (extreme severity)

This rating is applied when a symptom is sufficiently affecting the patient's general functioning so that intensive psychotherapeutic intervention is required. Institutionalization may or may not be utilized depending on other variables, such as the resources within the home environment.

Example: A patient suffers from psychogenic "stomach aches" which have kept him away from school with increasing regularity, and are currently averaging 2 days per week.

"6" RATING (incapacitating severity)

This rating is applied when a symptom has completely incapacitated the patient from functioning within the expected or usual societal structure appropriate to him. The severity of the symptom will disallow his either living at home or attending public school. With all symptoms rated "6," institutionalization is required.

Example: A patient's bizarre behavior, *i.e.,* homicidal attack of a classmate, has led to his permanent dismissal from public school and his being held by the department of corrections.

The GAP symptom list and Alpern's severity ratings have been used by the author and his colleagues in longitudinal follow-up investigations. Such ratings can readily be taught to non-professional, trained raters who would be unable to cope with the much more complicated diagnostic categories. In one study of 204 cases with a total of more than 1,000 symptoms, trained raters obtained a symptom selection and categorization agreement of 63.91%. Differences were resolved by discussion and consensus. An agreement of 73.2% was reached on the symptom severity ratings (study in process). The objectivication of such data will hopefully permit a comparison among the many variables which seem to have a relationship to the child's degree of health or disability at various times in the course of his treatment.

CLASSIFICATION OF A CASE IN WHICH THE PSYCHOPA-THOLOGY SEEMS NOT YET CRYSTALLIZED

Recall the case of Granville 9. (p. 148), the 7½-year-old black boy, who was very aggressive with other children and who was failing the first grade. Upon completion of the diagnostic study the staff concluded (p. 159), "Granville's problems at this time represent a behavior disorder which assumes the pattern of a characterological disorder. However, fixed patterns do not seem well established yet." Granville's case quite easily fits within "Unsocialized aggressive reaction of childhood" (308.4), DSM-II, p. 50. His symptoms were certainly not "transient" and yet the staff did not feel he was severe enough to warrant a "label" of personality disorder. According to GAP #62 we would categorize Granville in the following way:

> (3a) Developmental Deviation in Maturational Patterns; (5) social and (8) integrative development.
> Symptoms:
> (IIB) Learning Failure, 1.c. underachievement (severity rating "4")
> (IVB) Disturbed Maturational Patterns Development, delayed achievement of autonomy, poor impulse control and overactive use of denial and suppression (severity rating "5")
> (VA) Aggressive Behavior, 1. c.d.f., destructive, fighting and physical attacks (severity rating "5")

We prefer the GAP classification because it clearly specifies the impairment in social and integrative development and provides sufficient symptom description for comparison with the clinical picture at subsequent evaluations.

One final issue must be raised. Should a statement about the child's environment, usually his parents, be included in the nosological diagnosis? Even the thought of such an undertaking at this point in time is overwhelming. Nearly 20 years ago, Caplan[16] stressed that most of the world's child mental health workers recognize the whole family as a relevant field of focus. However, study of this important area is seriously impeded by lack of a framework against which we can define the effect of the family. The child's natural dependency makes it essential that his unique environment be studied thoroughly and this is reported in the diagnostic formulation. Those upon whom the child is dependent must be studied as possible contributors to the etiology. Even more importantly, the environment's ability to understand, sustain and cooperate with the treatment process is frequently a major element in choice of treatment and the prognosis.

Perhaps listing additional diagnoses from DSM-II for each important adult should be considered. In the case of Jeffrey M. with school refusal (pp. 129-148) his management and his prognosis would have been altered considerably if his mother were suffering a major psychosis and/or were seriously suicidal. However, frequently the parents of a child with a mental disorder do not show an identifiable or classifiable emotional or personality illness. There may be a frequently changing environment as was true for 2½-year-old R.T. (p. 69) who suffers seriously impaired development. How could one succinctly describe and classify the family situation of Granville A. (pp. 148-161)? Yet, in every case the milieu is crucial for diagnosis and treatment planning.

The author[68] and some of his colleagues have spent several years developing a "Parent Treatability" scale. The instrument appears valid in that several parental factors appear to be relevant to the guardian's ability to make changes in the child's environment. However, several years of clinical application will be necessary before even a guess can be made about the scale's usefulness within a disease classification system.

For the present we must content ourselves with including a description of the child's surroundings in the case formulation. Perhaps a parental assessment should not be a part of his statistical diagnosis. The issue is raised because of our conviction of the importance of the child's environment. If we are to advance our knowledge in this area it seems we must develop a method for dissecting and classifying specific elements in the child's living arena which are truly most relevant to his illness and his treatment.

SUMMARY

Learning to classify children's mental disorders has been resisted and neglected by clinicians. Yet, if a type of disability cannot be described and classified, it cannot be scientifically studied. An ideal classification system would clarify diagnosis and focus treatment. A generally accepted nomenclature is essential also for administrative and scientific reasons.

A practical nomenclature and classification system must evolve over time with continued clinical application. It must be revised as new knowledge develops. The APA, DSM-II (1968) is the most generally accepted nomenclature system in America today and it can be used for classifying children's disorders. However, this system is not specific enough for child psychiatry, is vague in differentiating "transient" conditions from the more classical neuroses and personality disturbances and it entirely neglects the disorders most accurately seen as developmental deviations.

Recognizing some shortcomings, the author recommends that child psychiatrists officially adopt GAP Report #62 for clinical and scientific use. With experience this latter system could hopefully be updated for inclusion in future revisions of the APA Diagnostic and Statistical Manual.

As long as our diagnostic categories remain primarily based upon descriptive phenomenology, the diagnosis needs to be clarified by a listing of the child's specific symptoms and the severity of these symptoms at any given point in time.

The GAP #62 symptom list and the Alpern Symptom Severity Rating Scale have proved most useful, particularly in long term follow-up of children.

The child's natural dependency make it essential that some evaluation of his environment be included in the diagnostic formulation and treatment planning. It is regrettable that so far we have no generally accepted method for describing and classifying crucial elements in the environment. Again, an entity cannot be scientifically studied until it can be objectively identified. Whether the environment can be classified with the child's diagnosis or must be separately classified may not be terribly important. However, the environment usually seems to be an integral part of the child's stability or instability and it seems incumbent upon us to seriously try to objectify our concepts of the family.

Chapter 10

TREATMENT

THE "case study" in outline or any other form does not automatically decide who should be treated and what the treatment should be. A thorough review of all forms of psychiatric treatment, including indications, contraindications, and techniques, is beyond the scope of this text. However, consideration of some of the general principles underlying the assessment of diagnostic data as it relates to treatment planning is in order. Decisions about treatment planning for any particular child are dependent upon the nature and severity of the impairment or disability, the causes of the disorder, and the prognosis.

In the still-developing individual, severity of disability is relative to the functioning of others of the same age group and to the effect of the current disability on the child's maturation. The experienced clinician uses empirical concepts to differentiate normalcy from abnormalcy at the various age levels and to prognosticate the future. Etiology must be considered in the light of the accumulated body of knowledge regarding the genesis of both normal and deviant development. Unless the clinician wishes to restrict his practice to a very narrow segment of childhood disorders, he must use an eclectic approach in assigning causes and planning treatment. Facts and theories about child development and symptom formation must be adapted to the case in hand. Case study formulations such as those presented on the preceding pages permit us to ask ourselves, "Which theoretical constructs about etiology and treatment are most applicable for this child?" The fact that the child is still undergoing the maturational process makes prognostication extremely difficult. We usually tread a narrow line between undertreatment and overtreatment of a specific situation or set of symptoms. Nevertheless, unwarranted optimism or a defeating pessimism on the part of the parents and the clinician has serious implications for the future of the child.

Even though severity of illness, etiology, and prognosis are interdependent, they must receive independent consideration in planning appropriate therapy. For example, a child with a moderate impairment of ego functioning can sometimes improve dramatically under a treatment program directed at his environment alone, if the illness has been of short duration and the environmental stress is amenable to change. However, another child equally ill may require quite different treatment if his illness has been of long duration and/or the noxious environmental circumstances are intractible. In the latter instance the child may require considerable individual psychotherapy to resolve old, established conflicts and unhealthy defenses and to find reasonably healthy compensatory mechansims. Such a child often needs special or remedial education to bring him educationally up to his peer group. An educational lag compounds a neurosis and often does not spontaneously disappear upon resolution of the neurosis unless the child is exceptional. For reasons not clearly understood, we also find children with relatively little disturbance in their current adjustment in spite of an emotionally chaotic environment. In these cases, treatment is aimed primarily at prevention of future illness rather than current maladaptations.

Since behavior, both normal and abnormal, is always multidetermined, it is quite difficult to avoid confusing our clinical observations with our theoretical constructs. This hazard for the clinician can be reduced if he will first decide on the basis of his examination the depth or degree of illness.

Theoretical considerations then become important in deciding which of the possible etiological factors are most relevant to that particular child's illness and by what method or methods the situation can be corrected or ameliorated.

SEVERITY OF THE ILLNESS

The degree of current malfunctioning is the first consideration. "How sick is sick?" and "How sick is this child?" are, in practice, rather abstract questions. In adult mental conditions, the severity of the illness is determined by the nature of the symptoms, the amount of suffering experienced by the patient, and the resultant interference with important functions. Anna Freud[20] points out that these criteria are not valid when applied to children. Psychological and behavioral symptomatology in children, especially the very young, changes from day to day, even from hour to hour. This phenomenon leaves both parents and trained observers wondering whether a particular piece of behavior is a temporary reaction to environmental and developmental stresses or a more permanent and crippling personality and behavioral deviation. For example, fire setting must always be taken seriously because of its consequences. However, such behavior may occur accidentally; it may be done by a preschool child who is inadequately supervised, by a child who is temporarily reacting to some acute environmental stress such as disruption of parental or parent-child relationships, by a child who is acting out some neurotic conflict, or by a child whose reality testing and judgment are impaired by psychotic thinking. Hence, even such serious behavior as fire setting does not alone establish the severity of the illness. If the act is done repeatedly, it is definitely some mental or emotional disturbance and not accidental, and a complete clinical examination of the child is necessary to determine the depth of the disturbance.

The amount of suffering or psychological distress experienced by the child patient may make him more willing to submit himself to treatment, but it does not reflect the depth of his illness. Usually the parental suffering or anxiety is much greater than the child's. The child is apt to see his own suffering, if any, as secondary to the adults' reactions to him and not the result of his symptoms. Blandness in response to the normal stresses of growing up may be a symptom in itself.

Using the degree of impairment of functioning as a criterion of severity has similar limitations. There is no absolute prototype of the perfectly functioning child at any age level. Again, children's social functioning has a wide range of variability within the norm, and fluctuation in the level of performance is typical of the developmental process.

Anna Freud[26] states that impairment of the child's capacity to move forward in progressive steps until maturation and development are completed is the only reliable indicator of the severity of the illness. Emotionality is a part of normal growing up, but emotional upsets must be taken seriously if development is arrested, slowed up, or reversed.

Sabshin[62] reminds us that the evaluation of treatment and of preventive programs depends upon our concept of normality. At present there is insufficient empirical data from a variety of populations to test our normative hypotheses properly. What he calls "normality as process" stresses that "normal behavior is the end result of interacting systems that change over time." Society's acceptance of what is normal is subject to evolutionary modification, as statistical averages, the range of health, and ideal values all change with the passage of time. Just as time and chance are the essential elements of Sabshin's favored approach to the concept of normal behavior, the *capacity* to progress developmentally over time is the crux of the child's relative state of psychological health or illness.

Of course, this should not mean we must wait until the patient has reached maturity before it can be determined whether his illness was serious or not. As was stated, the situation is serious if the patient's development is slowed up, reversed, or arrested. It is necessary then to determine whether the developmental impairment is only partial or nearly complete; that is, whether only a few or many facets of the personality are affected. We feel that the degree of developmental impairment can be determined by a qualitative and quantitative assessment of the ego functions.

RELATION OF SEVERITY OF ILLNESS TO ULTIMATE PROGNOSIS

While the seriousness of the illness is relevant to the child's future, it is not synonymous with prognosis. Prognosis is an estimate of whether or not the child can resume forward movement toward complete maturation. It depends upon many things, such as whether factors within the child or his environment are still operating to interfere with maturation. Are these etiological agents subject to eradication in whole or in part? If the causes can be removed, is the organic or psychological damage reversible? What is the child's ability to compensate for certain deficits in his ego functioning? In the case of an adult whose social role, vocational achievement, and behavior patterns are well established, it is somewhat easier to estimate outcome or establish goals of therapy. We review the adult's premorbid adjustment and the extent to which it has been affected by the illness. With this information the adult's therapist has at least some guideposts for prognostication. Since children are still evolving physically, chronologically, and socially, they provide us with few criteria for estimating the ultimate potential of their ego capacities and their ability to compensate for functional deficits.

In therapy, child psychiatrists expect the growth potency to assist in the healing process. However, without some adequate measure of these potentials, they are unreliable for treatment planning. In short, you hope the child's youth will assist recovery but you don't count on it completely. Pinpointing the "severity or seriousness of illness" in terms of the adequacy of ego functions at the time of examination helps decide whether treatment should be directed at strengthening or relaxing the internal and external controls, at improving peer or adult relations, at resolving neurotic conflicts, at developing a broader repertoire of defense mechanisms, at progressing from primary to secondary process thinking, or at compensating for unalterable ego deficiencies. Treatment planning may include one or many of these goals, which must be attained through direct therapy of the child as well environmental manipulation.

Establishing goals of therapy as outlined should be possible for each child, but such precise pinpointing of aims is seldom easy. Selecting the most appropriate form or methods of therapy is no simple matter either. In the introduction to her book, Haworth[35] speaks of the "still-nascent state" of child therapy. It is too early to write a definitive text on child psychiatric therapy, and only a few broad, general principals can be stated regarding adapting specific therapies to various childhood mental and emotional disorders. Many forms of therapy are still being clinically tested and validated. We are also faced with the overwhelming problems of multiple causation and great variability from child to child.

Psychotherapy for one or more members of the family has been the main treatment offered to date. There is no one psychotherapeutic model which will fit all conditions of children. Not only is the exact process of psychotherapy determined by the theoretical persuasion of the therapist, but it should be modified and adapted to the exact nature of the patient's problems. Today, the child therapist must be acquainted with a reasonable variety of individual psychotherapeutic techniques. He must also comprehend the values and pitfalls of counseling and/or therapy for parents, of group therapy for a variety of ages and conditions, of family group therapy, of remedial education, of child placement, and of our most recently acquired drug therapies.

It is most likely that each of these therapies has some usefulness for some, but not all, child psychiatric conditions. Through clinical experience during training and subsequent practice, clinicians learn empirically to select and vary therapy to suit the nature of the children's illnesses. The problems of scientifically matching and validating the selection of specific forms of treatment to particular childhood disorders are in need of immediate vigorous research effort. However, utopian scientific accuracy in the treatment process is an unrealistic expectation. Clinical judgment is essential for treatment planning and execution.

Basic principles of therapy can be learned from the literature. Several references are listed in the introduction of this book. However, the endless number of variables to be encountered in the therapeutic processes with different children cannot be satisfactorily described on the printed page. It is not likely that textbooks or other teaching devices can supplant supervised clinical training in the foreseeable future. It is incumbent upon the student to sharpen his diagnostic skills and recognize pathology in order to comprehend more readily the instructions of his preceptors in the intricate processes of therapy.

SUMMARY

There are many varieties of psychiatric disorders in children. Sharpening diagnostic skills, especially in defining the nature and depth of the illness, will improve one's ability to select the most effective treatment program for any given child. Spontaneous remission of symptoms commonly occurs in children. It is, therefore, not essential to treat vigorously every emotional upset of a child. He may be considered emotionally ill if his development is slowed up, arrested, or reversed. If such maturational impairments are not likely to remit spontaneously, treatment is indicated.

In planning treatment the clinician must pinpoint the areas of the personality that are most severely affected and the degree or severity of the impairment. He must then decide if the causes of the child's personality deviation are reversible or not. If the causes are removed, can the child be expected to resume normal development or is the damage to the personality so severe that rehabilitative and compensatory measures will be required?

The wide variety of currently available treatment methods are listed. The problems of multiple causation and high variability of response from child to child make it essential that treatment be learned by clinical practice under close supervision of an experienced preceptor. A diagnostic formulation based upon a thorough study of the child and his family is the starting point for treatment. As new knowledge is learned about the patient or changes occur in him during treatment, the formulation and treatment program can be appropriately altered.

Chapter 11

CONSULTATIONS

In the foregoing chapters we reviewed examination techniques as a part of the diagnostic evaluation and treatment planning. The examination of children for the specific purpose of advising other professionals, *i.e.* consultation, is much the same but has some definite differences. When a child comes or is brought to us for treatment our primary responsibility is to that patient and his parents. However, in consultation our primary responsibility is to the consulter. Unless or until the consulter, the consultant, and the family mutually agree that the consultant shall take complete charge of the case, the consultant is advisor to the consulter and the consulter remains directly responsible to and for the patient. Adhering to this principle is not blindly accepting traditional medical ethics or etiquette. Patients can be rendered serious disservice when consulter-consultant roles are confused. For example, there may be misunderstanding about who is taking the responsibility for reviewing the findings and recommendations with the responsible adults to the end that nothing is done for the child. Families frequently complain they were told nothing after rather extensive evaluation procedures. We fear that all too often this complaint is justified. Equally serious from the patient's standpoint are those instances in which the consultant and consulter have misunderstandings or honest differences of opinion and the family is given confusing or contradictory advice.

When a colleague refers a patient for diagnosis and treatment or it is mutually decided the consultant should take complete responsibility for a case, the above problems do not occur. However, such situations are not appropriately termed "consultation" in its strictest meaning. For purposes of this discussion, we define consultation as a situation in which one professional, the consultant, is asked to give advice to another professional, the consulter, about a third party called "the patient". The consulter already has some professional relationship with the patient but is not the parent or personal guardian of the child. There is not the customary doctor-patient relationship but a patient-consulter-consultant relationship. A complete diagnostic evaluation may be necessary but the child psychiatrist consultant may be limited to addressing himself to specific questions raised by the consulter. The situation that most closely meets our definition of consultation is when the consulter asks for suggestions related to his specific role with a child. A teacher might seek advice regarding classroom management or remedial procedures for a learning problem. A social worker may wish help in selecting a placement or a physician may ask for consultation regarding the emotional concomitants of medical management. In each of these examples the child psychiatrist does not execute his own recommendations. The effectiveness of his advice is dependent upon the comprehension and clinical skills of the consulter as well as the advisor's diagnostic acumen. The consultant must be truly skilled in diagnosing and prognosticating. His recommendations must not only offer the best possible solutions for the questions asked, but dare not involve technical feats which are beyond the time, motivation, or skill limitations of the consulter. The consulter-consultant relationship is a crucial interaction to which we will return with more details later.

THREE TYPES OF CONSULTATION SERVICES

We have used an individual case, problem-centered definition of the consultation process which is appropriate in many service settings. However, recognition must be given to other forms of consultation such as participation in program planning with community groups and child caring agencies. Advice may be sought regarding the design and implementation of clinical services for a particular population or regarding the preventive potential of various non-clinical projects or programs being planned for children. Caplan[17] clearly states the philosophy behind this type of consultation, "A community focus does not entail neglect of the individual, but rather a wider responsibility, not only for the welfare of those individuals who happen to be currently visible because they have come for help, but also for the others of which these are but a sample." This kind of consultation is appropriate for private and public health, education and welfare agencies but is usually not requested by individual practitioners.

A third type of consultant role requires teaching and administrative skills to assist a variety of medical and non-medical children's agencies with in-service training programs and staff coordination problems. Requests for this type of service usually come from established agencies with trained and experienced staff who wish to upgrade the quality of their services. The consultant may give formal lectures and seminars, assist the administrator in employee selection and with personnel problems, or even offer individual and group counseling sessions designed to enhance the personal and professional effectiveness of the staff. Similar types of assistance may also be desired by various professional training schools. In these latter instances, the child psychiatrist may be considered a member of the part-time faculty rather than a consultant. Even if the primary assignment is teaching, most service agencies or institutions also expect their consultant to give advice on individual cases and assist in carrying out treatment plans for some children.

CONSULTATIONS IN NON-MEDICAL SETTINGS

The teaching-consultant role is a most gratifying one for many child psychiatrists. It is enjoyable to share one's knowledge and skills with a group of sophisticated people who are eager to learn. We also believe we can make a much greater, long range impact on the welfare of many more children by improving the skills of other professionals than by individual case treatment. This is truly primary prevention with the aim of reducing the actual incidence of developmental and mental disorders in a given population or secondary prevention which is early case finding to prevent the progression to serious or intractable disability. Prevention on a mass basis is an ideal to which we can aspire. However, in practice, most consulters need and usually request individual case-oriented assistance. The staff of many institutions and schools are overwhelmed with the most serious types of problems. They desperately want relief from the pressure of their most burdensome children. They may resent the time required and the implications about their own skills if the consultant insists on being only their pedagogue. After the consultant has demonstrated his skills with individual cases, he can hope requests for teaching his skills will be forthcoming. Some child psychiatrists also resist the expansion of the consultant's role beyond that of individual case management. It is incumbent upon the consultant to be constantly sensitive to the immediate needs of the consulter. He dare not assume that he knows what is best for others who wish his help. Failure to have the consultation aims and the functions of the consultant clearly defined can result in a breakdown of the consultation process and thus deprive some children of needed services.

Most adults who take care of groups of children sooner or later become concerned with primary and secondary prevention of mental and emotional disabilities. This reflects a sincere interest in the quality of life for children and a realistic acceptance that there will never be enough trained psychiatric persons to treat all who need it. This mutual interest in prevention accounts for the fact most child psychiatrists spend a significant amount of their time working with schools, placement services, and correctional institutions. Many of the concepts now included under the rubric, "Community Psychiatry" have emanated from these consultation practices. There is ample literature on the subject of agency consultations and it will not be discussed further in this text. The reader is referred to the work of Berkovitz,[14] Caplan,[16,17] and Krugman[44] for theoretical background and practical examples of consultation in non-medical settings.

RELATIONS OF CHILD PSYCHIATRISTS WITH MEDICAL COLLEAGUES

The consulter-consultant relationship can be extremely sensitive and fragile in hospitals and clinics. Around the country the relationships among family physicians, pediatricians and child psychiatrists are quite variable. The degree of communication among these specialties is so vital to the consultation process that a close inspection of the current state of affairs is certainly warranted.

Some family physicians and pediatricians seldom, if ever, ask for a psychiatric consultation. This may be the result of the unavailability of psychiatrists or lack of confidence in the psychiatrist's abilities. It is doubtful if there are any physicians in America today who do not know that the subspecialty of child psychiatry exists. However, child psychiatrists are comparatively few in number and there are many doctors in practice who have never personally met one of us. They often assume with some validity that child psychiatrists exist only in large metropolitan centers, are inundated with referrals, and barricaded behind long waiting lists. Certainly, this was universally true until just the past few years and is still true in many parts of the country. Many physicians are reluctant to put their patients through the time and expense required for psychiatric care, especially if the doctor has had no experience working with this newest of subspecialties and does not know if it will be truly helpful to his patient.

When a member of our specialty enters a medical community that has not previously had the services of a child psychiatrist, he will find that many laymen and a few medical colleagues are eager for his services and may even have unrealistic expectations of him. However, many of the medical profession, at least in more conservative communities, are apt to be skeptical or even rejecting. The most palatable explanation of this predicament is to assume that our non-psychiatric colleagues are prejudiced. Such projection does not solve the problem.

It cannot be denied that biases against psychiatry do exist. Improving the quantity and quality of psychiatric teaching in undergraduate and postgraduate medical education is reducing and hopefully will eventually eliminate erroneous attitudes. In the meantime, the posture and behavior of the child psychiatric consultant can either strengthen or ameliorate negative attitudes toward our subspecialty.

HOW CAN THE CHILD PSYCHIATRIST CONSULTANT BEST SERVE HIS MEDICAL COMMUNITY?

Many psychiatry training programs and national funding agencies deprecate the individual case approach. They rationalize that it is only "shoveling sand against the tide" and unless we teach our medical colleagues in primary and secondary prevention we can never hope to make an impact upon the overwhelming amount of mental disorder among children. The other side of the argument is that unless we make friends with our colleagues and provide concrete demonstrations that our clinical skills can be effective, we will have little opportunity to teach them anything at all. The majority of physicians are more conservative than psychiatrists. They are apt to subscribe to the adage that "those who can, 'do' and those who can't do, 'teach'". Rightly or wrongly the average physician has been trained and constantly admonished to provide direct clinical service. He deserves our assistance with the most serious psychiatric problems in his practice. Traditionally, he has received this kind of help from other medical specialists and he finds the psychiatrist, who shuns direct patient responsibility but is ever willing to advise others about how to improve patient care, a complete enigma.

This argument about whether the child psychiatrist consultant in a medical setting can use his time more wisely by teaching his special skills to other physicians or by adopting the modus operandi of the traditional medical consultant can only be understood if it is viewed in historical perspective. It is a paradox that although child psychiatrists are by definition trained in medicine and in psychiatry, the practice of child psychiatry did not originate in medical schools nor in psychiatric centers and hospitals. Except for the care of the mentally retarded and severely psychotic, few psychiatrists were involved with the treatment of children prior to the turn of this century. As a part of the "American Mental Hygiene Movement" or perhaps as a by-product of the "Movement" some psychiatrists became consultants to juvenile courts, schools, child welfare and other agencies. William Healy is perhaps the best known of many who participated in the origins of child psychiatry as a specialty. Child guidance clinics developed within courts and schools and later as autonomous, community-supported agencies separate from the mainstream of medicine and psychiatry. The overwhelming demand for service, the slowness in development of large numbers of trained manpower and the dedication to long, arduous individual treatment caused the notorious "waiting list" and only further isolated the child psychiatrist from his medical colleagues. Child psychiatrists have been admonished to give up the individual case approach and dedicate their efforts to teaching their skills to medical colleagues and paramedical personnel. In the extreme this is unrealistic. The child psychiatrist must keep considerable patient responsibility if he is to maintain his own clinical skills, have continued awareness of his shortcomings, and be accepted as a practicing clinician. However, he must also be willing and able to teach those who can and are willing to learn from him.

There is a trend in all of medicine away from the individual treatment of disease toward prevention and health maintenance. The child psychiatric consultant must avail himself of every opportunity to practice as well as teach the principles of early treatment and prevention. However, too much zeal in changing the traditional medical consultant model often conveys a messianic attitude and can be self-defeating in the long run. Idealistic goals of teaching our clinical skills to others and involving our colleagues in primary and secondary prevention of mental illness can best be achieved if we are willing to demonstrate the efficacy of our knowledge in the traditional clinical setting of the generalist and other specialists. We, as specialists, must always remain willing to carry a major share of responsibility for psychiatrically ill children. It is unrealistic and condescending to expect all other physicians to handle "the minor" psychiatric problems or those persons with a poor prognosis. Many physicians cannot and should not treat psychiatric problems. They will remain dependent upon us for the treatment of all or most of the psychological disorders that appear in their practice for the same reasons we need them to treat the physical ills of our patients. Fortunately, there is an increasing number of physicians who want us to teach them how to manage mental disorders in their own hospitals and offices. The child psychiatrist consultant must be willing to teach other professionals and also to render a considerable amount of direct patient service.

THE CONSULTANT IN A PEDIATRIC TEACHING HOSPITAL

While nearly all medical institutions are committed to service, teaching, and research, none or very few have the funds or available talent to perform each of these activities in equal quantity and with comparable quality. In a private practice sector there will be emphasis upon direct clinical service with precious little monies or staff time for teaching and research. In a setting where teaching commitments are backed up with budget, direct service demands are usually less. The world needs both so we cannot say that one setting is more socially useful than the other. The important point is that the consultant be aware of the real expectations of the particular medical community in which he is working. In a setting committed to teaching, the consultant can expect gradually over the years to devote more time to informal and formal teaching and less to direct patient care. When working with colleagues who are service oriented and carrying heavy case loads, the consultant will probably have little time for teaching beyond that which is incidental to patient care.

From the long range standpoint, the consultant's time is most effectively utilized in a setting where he can render some direct clinical services and still put special emphasis on teaching his colleagues child psychiatric principles and techniques. Peer review systems are rapidly becoming a reality and re-examination for licensure and re-certification will soon be a regular part of professional life. These two factors will make continuing education mandatory and will force all medical facilities and communities to make teaching activities a significant budgetary item. Therefore, it seems appropriate here to review consultation procedures in the clinical teaching medical situation.*

The three essential elements of a consultation service are (1) prompt service, (2) effective communication to clarify the immediate problems, and (3) adequate follow-through of realistic recommendations. This means that there can be no waiting list; the consulter and consultant must have direct verbal interchange to reach agreement on the problems needing attention at once; and, definitive treatment services must be readily available when necessary. In-hospital consultation patients must be seen the same day the request is received or within 24 hours. Consultations on out-patients often must be seen immediately, but some can be scheduled. Not all consultation requests are of an emergency nature but the consulter and the family are usually unwilling and unable to wait for answers to their questions. Being available to offer immediate consultation risks reducing the quality of service and making the third essential, "adequate follow-through", an impossibility. The following description of consultation procedures will illustrate how these pitfalls can be avoided.

---

*The procedures described and the case examples are from the Child Psychiatry Consultation Service of Riley Children's (general pediatrics) Hospital, Indiana University School of Medicine. Modifications to fit other hospitals will obviously be necessary.

THE PROCESS OF CONSULTATION IN A MEDICAL SETTING

When fellows in child psychiatry training are first assigned to the consultation service, they are overwhelmed with the demand for service and complain bitterly about "inappropriate" referrals. Since all physicians are taught to request a consultation if his patient's problem is beyond his level of competence, it seems there can be no such thing as an "inappropriate" consultation request. Consultations are most often requested on the most complex types of cases. The trainee-psychiatrist feels he simply cannot do justice to the many questions about the case and still keep his time free to respond immediately to the next consultation request. The consultant must accept certain limitations of his role if he is to be readily available to see new cases. He cannot and should not do a complete diagnostic study including detailed history, psychological testing, and mental status as portrayed in Chapter 10. He will not be able to find definitive answers to all of the child's problems. His most important function is one of "triage." With the aid of his own mental status examination and as much personal and family history as he can get quickly, he must answer the following questions in this order: (1) How seriously ill is this child? (2) How urgent is it that some definitive diagnosis and treatment plans be made? (3) Are there any immediate measures that ought to be tried to relieve the urgency of the situation? (4) What is the next logical step toward sound and first-rate psychological care for this child? The consultant must stick to pragmatic issues and strongly resist the temptation to completely unravel every provocative facet of every case.

The consulter's questions are often not clear on the consultation note or phone message. Some examples of bewildering referral questions or statements are: "Johnny Jones is on Ward R. Please evaluate." "Dr. B. wishes psychometrics (mental measurements) on Mary Smith." "Billy Z. was admitted 3 days ago with c.c. of 'x' and 'y'. Please advise if the etiology is functional or organic." "There is a bad family situation and the child is in need of immediate psychiatric care."

"On rounds yesterday Dr. A., the chief of service, said a psychiatric evaluation should be done before the child is discharged. The child was admitted 18 days ago. All studies are completed and we would like to discharge him this afternoon." Such referrals reveal a profound naivete about emotional disorders and psychiatric procedures. They may also be ego deflating for the psychiatrist. These are extreme examples chosen for illustrative purposes. Many referral requests do clearly indicate what specific kind of help the consulter needs. In any event, it is imperative that the consultant confer directly with the consulter to find out what facts about the patient led to the request for psychiatric evaluation and how it is anticipated that the psychiatrist's opinion will be helpful. Does the conferring doctor want the consultant to take over the total management of the case?; offer psychiatric therapy concomitant with the physical treatment?; or merely offer advice on how the primary physician can provide total care himself? The answers to these questions are determined mutually by both physicians. In the majority of instances, the consulter-physician does not want advice. Even those most sympathetic with child psychiatry's manpower problems hope the consultant will accept the patient for definitive care.

A reliable history is an essential part of any medical work up. With rare exceptions consultants of all specialties take their own history to be certain that questions relative to their area of special interest are covered. The psychiatrist is fortunate if the hospital has social service workers who can obtain a good social developmental history, important information which does not appear routinely in medical charts. If such social service help is available, he may then only have to briefly meet the parents to be certain he has informed consent to examine their child and to offer them any reassurances they may need about himself and his profession before proceeding to examine the child.

A mental status examination of the child is essential in every instance. Serious errors occur when advice is given with only a sparse second-hand history and without personally seeing the child. However, as stated before, the consultant cannot always do a complete diagnostic study. It is sufficient to have a brief family-social history and a partial mental status examination to determine the seriousness and urgency of the situation, and to decide if the complex nature of the problem warrants complete psychiatric study and treatment or if the primary physician and the consultant should enter into a short-term coordinated treatment program. The "triage" or "sorting" process is to distinguish which children need immediate and extensive evaluation and treatment in a psychiatric clinic or institution, which children need other types of child care or treatment services and which children can be helped with short-term or modified psychiatric procedures.

IDENTIFYING CASES FOR INTENSIVE PSYCHIATRIC CARE

Probably 60% or more of the children referred are suffering from chronic, multiple, mental, social and psychological problems. The primary or consulter physician may have been struggling for a long time to try to help the child and family, or he may have just recently become aware of the fact the child is seriously in need of psychological help. In either event the consultant and the consulter are now prepared to formulate and answer some immediate pragmatic questions. Some examples of these kinds of questions are: Where can we obtain definitive help for this child? Does he need out-patient treatment, residential treatment, psychiatric hospitalization, a remedial education program and/or placement out of the home? How can parental resistance to accepting psychiatric help be overcome? The child may have been seen previously by many social, medical and psychological agencies yet never been involved in a truly definitive type of treatment program. There is always the danger that a child with a mental disorder or with serious family social problems will "fall between the cracks," so to speak, in the maze of services available in the community. The consultant's knowledge of community resources and his ability to deal with family resistances are the skills needed by the consulter in these instances.

If repeated out-patient visits are needed, the family should be referred, if possible, to a psychiatric treatment center no more than 1 hour commuting time from their home. Transportation time and inconvenience are significant causes for "drop-outs" from all mental health clinics. It is best if the consulter, consultant and social worker can have a joint conference with the parents to recommend continued psychiatric study, to inform the parents of the facilities in their geographic location and try to deal with any apparent parental resistance. Ideally, the family should not merely be referred to their local agency but should be placed in *contact* with them. For some overburdened or unsophisticated parents it is necessary to involve local welfare or public health nursing services to assist in the follow-through. The consultant must have a practice or be affiliated with a clinic which will provide definitive psychiatric care for those in his geographic proximity. The same principles apply to childern who are retarded or suffering learning disabilities. Not infrequently, we have learned during the course of the consultation that the family is already involved in a treatment or rehabilitation program in their local school or community. A telephone call to the home community as well as discussion with the parents is needed to ascertain whether the family should be encouraged to continue with the local agency and whether there are any special questions the local professionals would wish to ask the consultant.

When our preliminary consultation indicates that the child will probably have to be placed out of the home, either because of his illness or the family situation, a complete diagnostic study may be necessary. Such a serious and potentially hazardous decision cannot be made lightly. In these instances the consultant must himself do a complete study or arrange that such a study be done at a facility convenient for the family.

SHORT TERM PSYCHIATRIC TREATMENT

The above described time-limited involvement and rapid disposition of the serious and chronic problems are necessary to keep the consultation unit from becoming bottlenecked. However, the consultant should provide treatment himself or in collaboration with the primary physician for patients suffering acute stress reactions and when psychological symptoms are a complication of a serious medical problem or are interfering with medical management. The variety of these cases are infinite.

The younger the child, the more vulnerable he is to environmental stress and the more likely it is that his anxiety will manifest itself in some type of somatic symptom. The most common such symptoms are feeding or sleep disturbances, abdominal pain, prolonged vomiting, regression in toilet training, acute phobias, malaise, sudden onset of tantrums and negativism, or acute onset of apathy and withdrawal. If the child's development up until the onset of symptoms has been reasonably normal, the family seems to have had relative stability and a stressful event has recently occurred, immediate trial of short term treatment is indicated. In many instances explanation of the psychological nature of the symptoms, plus revealing the connection between the symptoms and the stressful events during a few counseling sessions with the parents and child, will be sufficient. Should a few counseling sessions not resolve the problem or during the course of counseling serious psychopathology in the child or family become apparent, arrangements for more intensive psychiatric study and treatment will, of course, be necessary.

Frequently, young children with psychosomatic symptoms are reacting to a mild to moderate depression in one or both parents. In fact, this situation is so common that we routinely inquire about symptoms of depression and conscious, self-recognized melancholy in the parents. Busy house officers seldom recognize subtle signs of depression in the parent or discount such signs as normal "concern about the child." Parents almost never volunteer information about their own psychic health, especially if they are depressed. However, after open discussion they can often readily see the connection between their own moods and the onset or fluctuations of the child's symptoms.

Referral of the parent or parents for psychiatric treatment must be explored diplomatically and preferably should be a decision made mutually by the parent himself or herself, and the child's physician after review of the depth and seriousness of the depression or other illness in the parent. It is especially important for the pediatrician to be alert to prolonged or disabling postpartum depression. Such depression, when untreated, not only can result in physiological disturbances in the infant, but can have long-range detrimental effects upon the mother-child relationship. Medical students and young house officers usually look upon the well-baby clinic as a "boring chore". No doubt this is due to the heavy emphasis during medical school upon the intrigue of unusual and exotic pathologic conditions. Many students resist being taught the golden opportunity for primary prevention that exists in the neonatal and infant clinics. By contrast we have found the nurse-clinicians who now staff many well-baby clinics are most eager to learn the psycho-social-physiological approach to providing comprehensive care and prophylaxis for young families. The child psychiatrist consultant can teach them the interviewing techniques used in uncovering any psychosocial problems which are causing symptoms or interfering with the baby's development. These nurses are frequently quite adept in parental counseling and are most open to learning the judicious use of community agencies for helping troubled families.

PSYCHIATRIC TREATMENT IN CONJUNCTION WITH MEDICAL MANAGEMENT

As stated above, it is unfair and unrealistic to expect the nonpsychiatric physician to provide the treatment for children with serious and chronic mental disorders. The consultant must be prepared to provide this service or arrange that it be provided. On the other hand, short-term psychological treatment and prophylactic care may be provided by the primary physician, the consultant, or other hospital staff depending upon the circumstances and staff abilities. When a child requires both medical and psychiatric therapy the consultant has the opportunity to provide a unique and interesting type of patient service. These cases also provide a focus around which a maximum of mutual teaching and learning will occur between the consultant and consulter. These patients give the child psychiatrist many occasions to learn some of the recent advances in general medicine. Psychosomatic medicine is no longer a "game" of deciding functional versus organic causes of disease. We now must comprehend the unique and often subtle interdigitation of functional and organic elements influencing the symptoms and course of many illnesses. Although the nonpsychiatric physician may have little interest in mental disorders *per se,* he is almost invariably interested in comprehending psychological factors which are contributing to or complicating the management of physiological illnesses. Many of these physicians not only desire our assistance in treatment, but want to learn psychiatric techniques that they can use themselves in their regular practice. It is important that the pediatrician and family physician learn these treatment techniques because there simply are not enough child psychiatric man-hours to supply this kind of service. Even more important than manpower shortage is the fact that the patients (and especially parents) often will accept help with their psychological problems from the doctor in charge of the medical management more readily than from a psychiatrist. This may seem paradoxical yet it is true for several reasons. Discussing personal, emotional problems with the general medical doctor is easier because the "psychiatric stigma" is less or absent; there is an already established physician-patient relationship which is the major tool of psychotherapy and the patient can usually feel more confident that his "organic" problems will not be overlooked. Again, however, the decision about whether the consultant will be a co-therapist or an advisor to the primary therapist must be made by mutual agreement between the two physicians.

There are three broad categories of techniques appropriate to the psychiatric management of children already in treatment for some physiological condition: (1) The "search" for stresses or other causes, (2) therapeutic counseling of the child and his parents and (3) amelioration of symptoms even when the dynamics or causes cannot be immediately comprehended or definitively treated. The so-called "search for causes" is the beginning phase of therapeutic counseling. First and foremost the physician must learn the amount of psychic stress the child, the mother, and the father are each experiencing regarding the physical illness. The amount of psychic stress experienced by the patient may have little or no relationship to the seriousness of the illness as viewed by the objective mind of the medically trained person. Each of the principals (mother, father and child) should be asked to tell what they know of the illness, its cause, treatment, and its outlook. Next, other areas of the child's and family's life must be explored for foci of stress. Finally, one must always consider physiological or pharmacological factors as a cause of psychiatric symptoms.

Therapeutic counseling consists of trying to remove the actual stress or reducing its potency. Such counseling can be relatively brief and simple or may require prolonged work with the family. Nearly every illness produces some psychic stress which causes new emotional symptoms or exaggerates pre-existing ones. This is most evident in chronic disabilities and life-threatening illnesses. One can often predict the amount of assistance the family will need if he understands their characteristic ways of handling stress. Intensive counseling about the primary organic illness is needed for nearly all chronic illnesses and developmental problems. Many physicians seem to have a natural talent for interviewing and doing this type of counseling. These consulters will merely wish the consultant's reassurance that they are dealing with a stress reaction and that some additional, more serious, psychiatric disorder is not present. Other consulters will wish the consultant to do the counseling for them. Alternatives for counseling by the medical and psychiatric staff are, of course, the social service staff and various lay organizations such as Ostomy Clubs, groups for paralytics, cystic fibrosis, retardation, and other organizations which offer families assistance. In cases where the child is suffering a psychiatric disorder of a deeper nature than a reaction to his organic illness or certain character traits of the parents of the child make them inaccessible to counseling or if serious social problems exist, the consultant must provide or arrange for more intensive psychiatric or social work treatment which the attending physician usually cannot provide. The reader should understand that the "triage" and decision-making responsibility may remain with the consultant over a protracted period of time.

There are times when one may wish to try to remove psychological or behavioral symptoms by the use of pharmacological agents, hypnosis, or environmental manipulation. These measures are expedient and often humanitarian. Research reported by Nurnberger[58] recently has failed to confirm the belief that symptom removal without "insight" has a high risk of producing additional or more serious psychological or social symptoms. Rapid amelioration of symptoms can be problematic in that it is like "grasping in the dark" and too often doesn't work. When acute symptoms do disappear, it can be dramatic and gratifying, but also may lessen the motivation for more extensive psychiatric exploration and treatment of serious but less obvious or troublesome mental disturbances.

A few case examples will illustrate the points outlined above:

Psychological Treatment by the Primary Physician

It is the prerogative and responsibility of the attending physician and his team to treat or arrange for the treatment of the psychological symptoms that appear so often secondary to such illnesses as cardiac disease, diabetes, blood dyscrasias, retardation, postsurgical handicaps, congenital deformities, the dying child and many other illnesses which will require indefinite medical management. The consultant assists by helping the consulter sort out cases which are so serious or complicated that they are unlikely to respond to the limited time and expertise available to the consulter and his staff. However, through case conferences and seminars the consultant can help his medical and paramedical colleagues sharpen their counseling skills.

"Harry, age 13, was referred for psychiatric consultation because he had become uncooperative with follow-up treatment after removal of a malignant tumor and his mother reported temper tantrums and disobedience at home. The mental status examination was taped on TV and reviewed by the Child Psychiatry and Tumor Clinic staffs in conference.

"During the interview, Harry reviewed his many concerns about his siblings and his feelings about his father's desertion of the family several years ago. He also expressed considerable preoccupation with the amount of anxiety and the financial burden his illness had placed on his mother. Finally, after many indirect references, Harry was able to talk about his own fear of death. This was followed by ventilation of his anger related to the pharmacologic treatments which caused him 24 to 48 hours of physiological upset each time they were administered and he discussed his fear of re-hospitalization. He talked rather freely about his doctors, even though he knew the interview was being recorded for their review. He wanted to believe them, but was having great difficulty accepting their contention that his prognosis was good. Parenthetically, he expressed a dislike for all medical shows on TV except for Marcus Welby, where things always "turn out all right."

Following the case presentation and discussion, the consulter volunteered that he understood Harry better and would like to continue counseling the child himself with the psychiatric consultant's assistance.

"Mark, age 16, was referred by the Hematology Clinic because of profound depression and withdrawal. Mark had had many admissions and long experience with the hospital staff. His personality had changed drastically during the most recent exacerbation of his illness which was complicated by a nearly intractable lung infection. Mark was seriously ill but was able to come to the consultation office in a wheelchair and tolerated a 40-minute interview quite well. In contrast to Harry, Mark gave very little spontaneous information and denied all worries and all problems. He thought discussion of his future was useless and denied that he had ever even thought about the possibility that his leukemia might eventually be fatal. He understood the purpose of the interview, but stated that he had always found it was better not to talk about problems or unpleasant things. He requested that he not be forced to talk about things he didn't like and, specifically, that he not be required to have another psychiatric interview. This interview was also recorded on TV tape and reviewed in staff conference. During the discussion the hematology staff reported that shortly after the onset of his illness, Mark had been able to talk about the possibility of death and the poor prognosis for his illness. He had previously been seen as a cooperative and fairly outgoing young man. The staff was able to talk about their own frustration in trying to help him with his despair, but the final consensus was that we should respect his wishes and not force him to give up his denial and avoidance. His physician-in-charge and the chief nurse made arrangements for frequent visits to provide Mark with opportunities for ventilating his feelings and to give him reassurance of their continued interest and closeness, but not to force him to look at issues he was unable to face."

Similar types of case seminars demonstrating parental counseling have been used as a method of intensifying the counseling efforts of non-psychiatric clinics and services.

PSYCHOLOGICAL TREATMENT BY THE CONSULTING PSYCHIATRIST

Acute Hallucinosis

By mutual consent the consulting psychiatrist may take the major responsibility in the psychological management of physically ill children. Acute hallucinosis does not occur frequently but when it does it is most disturbing to the entire ward, the staff, and the family. At the present time these cases often remain an enigma to both the pediatrician and the psychiatrist. If the child has a history of previous psychosis or serious emotional disturbance, the stress of the hospitalization, the current illness or immediate circumstances may be the precipitating cause of the hallucinosis. In these cases the use of major tranquilizers and possibly psychiatric hospitalization may be necessary. In other patients without previous psychiatric history, we must consider that the hallucinosis may be the result of extreme stress or toxicity. These episodes seem to occur after serious burns, extensive surgery, or occasionally during a profound infection. The first step is to review all of the medications the child is receiving on the possibility of some untoward reaction to a particular medication or combination of drugs. In conference with the primary physician we try to reduce all medications to a minimum. If one suspects a toxic psychosis, one should be most cautious about adding any additional medications. General medical supportive measures are reviewed and the nursing staff and family are instructed in providing calm, continuous psychological support to the patient. These acute toxic hallucinatory episodes fortunately, in the author's experience, usually subside in a few days under good general supportive management.

Behavior Problems

"Tom, age 13, was referred by his orthopedic surgeon because of a behavior disorder which developed shortly after a diagnosis of spinal curvature was made and treatment was begun with a Milwaukee brace. Tom had begun failing in school, was irritable and disobedient around home. Both his pediatrician and his orthopedic surgeon had attempted to counsel Tom and were perplexed by his untoward reaction to the brace. The physicians' experience had been that most young people adjusted to this treatment quite well even though treatment might continue over many months.

"At the initial interview the psychiatrist asked Tom to tell him in his own words what he thought the problem was. Tom replied 'Well, doctor, I think you are going to find this a case of disturbed parent-child relationships'. Indeed, full study of the case indicated that there had been a long standing, subclinical disturbance in the parent-child relationships which had been worsened or been brought into focus by Tom's emotional upset in response to his orthopedic condition and treatment. This was a situation in which traditional child guidance therapy for both the parents and the child was indicated and was effective."

Reactions to Serious Handicaps

Paraplegics and quadraplegics are not referred for psychiatric consultation in any proportion to the actual incidence of the occurrence of these tragedies. Those who have been referred are usually extremely irritable, uncooperative with physical-medical rehabilitation treatment, unpleasant and disturbing to the ward staff, and upon psychiatric examination show signs of depression with an excessive use of denial of both psychological and physical signs. Treatment of these children is a major undertaking including intensive counseling of the parents, individual psychotherapy for the child and repeated conferences with the medical and rehabilitation staff as well as the nursing staff to arrange a therapeutic milieu or ward management type of program. The consultant can usually expect these patients to require a great deal of his time, but the psychological outcome can be most rewarding.

Removal of Symptoms

Relieving Anxiety with Medication

Some children are referred for acute anxiety which is so profound that it is painful for the staff, the family, and the psychiatrist to witness. Every effort is made to "search for the cause". In the interim, the use of tranquilizers in sufficient dosage to give the patient relief is certainly indicated.

Uses of Hypnosis

"Betty, age 14, was referred by the orthopedic staff because of violent outbursts and a combative response to even the most gentle physical therapy treatment of contractures in her lower limbs. At one point Betty struggled so hard the headboard fell off the bed. She would scream and cry violently when the physical therapist even approached her room. The parents and the physician were at their wits end. Psychiatric evaluation of Betty revealed a very histrionic personality in a girl who had been infantilized by her parents and was excessively dependent and demanding. She had no insight into how she alienated people and was extremely angry that no one would 'believe how terrible the pain is'. After two sessions of discussing with Betty the severity of her pain and yet the remaining need for physical therapy, the consultant talked with Betty about the possibility of trying hypnosis as a means of reducing her pain. Betty was agreeable to this and proved to be quite easily hypnotized. Shortly, she learned self-hypnosis and became amenable to the physical therapy under hypnosis. Following discharge from the hospital, further psychiatric evaluation and treatment was recommended to the family, but rejected."

Hypnosis or tranquilizers have also been found helpful for children with fatal illnesses and intractable pain in order to reduce the level of narcotic medication necessary.

Use of Behavior Modification

Consultation is frequently initiated by the nursing staff because of severe behavior problems on the ward. If the child must remain in the hospital for any length of time, it is important that a milieu therapy program be initiated. Many of these children have suffered long psychological and physical abuse and their family histories are replete with a wide variety of social and psychiatric illnesses. Sometimes transfer to a psychiatric residential treatment center is necessary. However, if this is not possible or not absolutely indicated, a therapeutic program within the general medical hospital can be initiated as an interim measure. This must be done by staff conference, including medical personnel, nursing, child-life workers, plus all other therapists and hospital personnel who will be taking part in the child's care and treatment while he is there. The principles of behavior modification are appropriately taught and applied in these situations.

The variety of cases encountered seems almost infinite. The above case material are only a few examples. Other psychiatrists, in other situations, might work with the same cases in different ways. However, irrespective of the setting and the inclinations of the consultant and consulter, the major issues are: to identify the problem, to identify its causes to the best of one's ability, decide upon an appropriate disposition or treatment and have a firm agreement regarding who will be responsible for expediting the plan. In formulating and carrying out treatment plans the first concern is for the welfare of the child. The extent to which we can involve house officers and others in actively designing and implementing these plans with us will determine how much we can teach them to use their own talents and the community's resources in alleviating children's psychological stresses and illnesses.

SUMMARY

Consultation is different from the usual diagnostic evaluation in several ways. The consultant's major responsibility is to the consulter rather than directly to the patient, and the urgency of the situation demands the psychiatrist act rapidly. The three types of consultation described are: (1) direct individual case consultation, (2) community planning of children's programs for primary and secondary prevention, and (3) teaching child psychiatric techniques to a wide variety of professionals who deal with the daily lives of children. The reader is referred elsewhere in the literature for instruction regarding consultation with community agencies and the major portion of this chapter is devoted to consultation in the medical setting.

The historical background of the apparent schism between child psychiatry and general medicine is reviewed. The actions of the child psychiatrist consultant may widen or lessen this schism. The traditional medical consultant model is recommended with the consultant acting as a "triage" center rather than personally offering definitive diagnosis and treatment for each case referred. Offering only time-limited service is necessary to prevent the consultant's schedule from becoming bottlenecked and a waiting list developing.

It is estimated that 60% or more of the cases referred have serious and profound psychiatric disorders. For these children the consultant's task is to assist the consulter and family in finding definitive psychiatric care. In the remainder of the cases, the child's psychiatric symptoms are the result of acute stress or the psychological disturbance is of such a nature that it is contributing to the total symptom picture or is interfering with the medical management of the illness. In these latter cases an immediate plan for either definitive or ameliorative psychiatric therapy must be made. Therapy will then be carried out by the consultant, by the primary physician with the consultant's guidance, or by non-medical professionals available in the hospital or the child's home community. A few case examples have been briefly presented to illustrate these various procedures.

Epilogue

Dr. Karl Menninger once told a class of residents that inability to translate our technical knowledge about a patient into plain English is a weakness of physicians in general and psychiatrists in particular. Menninger feels that the use of technical jargon often indicates a lack of complete understanding of the subject rather than the possession of superior knowledge. The author hopes this volume conveys the fact that psychiatric diagnosis and treatment planning for children is truly difficult but not beyond comprehension.

BIBLIOGRAPHY

1. Ackerman, N. W.: *Psychodynamics of Family Life.* New York, Basic Books, 1958.
2. Aichhorn, A.: *Wayward Youth.* New York, Viking Press, 1925, 1935, 1965.
3. Allen, F.: *Psychotherapy with Children.* New York, W. W. Norton & Co., Inc., 1942.
4. Allport, G. W.: *The Use of Personal Documents in Psychological Science.* New York, Social Science Research Council, 1942.
5. Alpern, G.: Personal Communication. Indiana University School of Medicine, 1973.
6. American Board of Psychiatry and Neurology, Inc.: Information for Applicants for Certification in Child Psychiatry; Rules and Regulations. 102 Second Avenue, S. W., Rochester, Minnesota, 1964.
7. American Psychiatric Association Research Report #18: *Diagnostic Classification in Child Psychiatry,* Jenkins and Cole (Eds.) Washington, D. C., 1964.
8. American Psychiatric Association Mental Hospital Service: *Diagnostic Statistical Manual for Mental Disorders.* Washington, D.C., 1952.
9. Ames, L., Learned, J., Metraux, R., and Walker, R.: *Child Rorschach Responses.* New York, Brunner-Mazel, 1974.
10. Ames, L., Metraux, R., and Walker, R.: *Adolescent Rorschach Responses.* New York, Brunner-Mazel, 1971.
11. Becker, W. C.: Consequences of Different Kinds of Parental Discipline, in *Review of Child Development Research,* Hoffman and Hoffman (Eds.) New York, Russell Sage Foundation, 1964, pp. 169–208.
12. Beiser, H. R.: Psychiatric Diagnostic Interviews with Children. *J. Amer. Acad. Child Psychiatry,* 1:656, 1962.
13. Beres, D.: Ego Deviations and the Concept of Schizophrenia, in *The Psychoanalytic Study of the Child.* New York, International Universities Press, Inc., 11:164, 1956.
14. Berkovitz, I. H. and Thomson, M.: Mental Health Consultation and Assistance to School Personnel of Los Angeles County. Los Angeles County Education Center, 9300 E. Imperial Highway, Downey, California 90242, 1973.

15. Berlin, I. N.: Book review in *Archives of General Psychiatry*, 22:575, 1970.
16. Caplan, G.: Recent Trends in Preventive Child Psychiatry, Chapter 7 in *Emotional Problems of Early Childhood*, G. Caplan (Ed.). New York, Basic Books, Inc., 1955, p. 153.
17. ————: *Principles of Preventive Psychiatry*. New York, Basic Books, Inc., 1964.
18. Chess, S.: *An Introduction to Child Psychiatry*, 2nd Ed. New York, Grune & Stratton, 1969.
19. Chess, S., Thomas, A., Birch, H.: Behavior Problems Revisited. *J. Amer. Acad. Child Psychiatry*, 6:321, 1967.
20. DeMyer, M. K., Barton, S., and Norton, J. A.: A Comparison of Adaptive, Verbal, and Motor Profiles of Psychotic and Nonpsychotic Subnormal Children. *Jour. Autism and Childhood Schizophrenia*, 2:359, 1972.
21. DeMyer, M. K., Norton, J. A. and Barton, S.: Social and Adaptive Behaviors of Autistic Children as Measured in a Structured Psychiatric Interview, unpublished paper.
22. Dodge, P. R.: Neurologic History and Examination, in *Pediatric Neurology*, T. W. Farmer (Ed.). New York, Harper & Row, 1964.
23. Ekstein, R.: Notes on the Teaching and Learning of Child Psychotherapy within a Child Guidance Setting. *Bulletin of the Reiss-Davis Clinic*, 3:68, 1966.
24. Erikson, E. H.: *Childhood and Society*. Rev. ed. New York, W. W. Norton & Co., 1964, pp. 209–246.
25. Finch, S. M.: *Fundamentals of Child Psychiatry*. New York, W. W. Norton & Co., Inc., 1960, pp. 37–44.
26. Freud, A.: *Normality and Pathology in Childhood*. New York, International Univ. Press, Inc., 1965, pp. 54–140.
27. ————: Regression as a Principle in Mental Development. *Bull. Menninger Clin.*, 27:126, 1963.
28. Freud, S.: *The Ego and the Id*. London, Hogarth Press, 1927, 1950, pp. 81–88.
29. Gildea, M., Glidewell, J. and Kantor, M.: Maternal Attitudes and General Adjustment in School Children; in *Parental Attitudes and Child Behavior*. Glidewell (Ed.). Springfield, Charles C Thomas, 1961, p. 89.
30. Goodenough, F. L.: *Measurement of Intelligence by Drawings*. New York, World Book Co., 1926.
31. Goodman, J., and Sours, J.: *The Child Mental Status Examination*. New York, Basic Books, 1967.
32. Group for the Advancement of Psychiatry Report No. 38: *The Diagnostic Process in Child Psychiatry*. New York, 1957, pp. 313–353.

33. Group for the Advancement of Psychiatry Report No. 62: *Psychopathological Disorders in Childhood; Theoretical Considerations and a Proposed Classification.* New York, 1966.
34. Hamilton, G.: *Psychotherapy in Child Guidance.* New York, Columbia University Press, 1947, pp. 34–44.
35. Haworth, Mary: *Child Psychotherapy,* New York, Basic Books, 1964.
36. Helper, M. M.: Parental Evaluations of Children and Children's Self-evaluations. *J. Abnorm. Soc. Psychol.,* 56:190, 1958.
37. Hirschberg, J. C. and Bryant, K. N.: Problems in the Differential Diagnosis of Childhood Schizophrenia, in *Neurology and Psychiatry in Childhood,* McIntosh and Hare (Eds.), Association for Research in Nervous and Mental Disease. Baltimore, The Williams & Wilkins Co., 1954, pp. 452–461.
38. Hunt, W. A., Wittson, C. L., and Hunt, E. B.: A Theoretical and Practical Analysis of the Diagnostic Process; in *American Psychopathological Association Proceedings,* New York, Grune & Stratton, 41:55, 1953.
39. Jackson, D. and Satir, V.: A Review of Psychiatric Developments in Family Diagnosis and Family Therapy; in *Exploring the Base for Family Therapy.* New York, Family Service Association of America, 1961, pp. 29–51.
40. Jessner, L. and Pavenstadt, E. (Eds.): *Dynamic Psychopathology in Childhood,* New York, Grune & Stratton, 1959.
41. Johnson, A. M. and Szurek, S. A.: The Genesis of Antisocial Acting Out in Children and Adults. *Psychoanal. Quart.,* 21: 323, 1952.
42. Klopfer, B. (Ed.): *Developments in the Rorschach Technique.* New York, World Book Co., 1956, pp. 3–44 and 88–180.
43. Koppitz, E.: *The Bender Gestalt Test for Young Children.* New York, Grune & Stratton, 1963.
44. Krugman, M. (Ed.): *Orthopsychiatry and the School.* New York, American Orthopsychiatric Association, 1958.
45. Ledwith, N.: *Rorschach Responses of Elementary School Children.* Pittsburgh, University of Pittsburgh Press, 1959.
46. Levitt, E. E.: A Comparison of Parental and Self-evaluations of Psychopathology in Children. *J. Clin. Psychol.,* 15:402, 1959.
47. ————: Psychotherapy Research and the Expectation-reality Discrepancy. *Psychotherapy: Theory, Research and Practice,* 3:163, 1966.
48. Lippman, H.: *Treatment of Children in Emotional Conflict.* 2nd ed. New York, McGraw-Hill Book Co., 1962.

49. Mark, J. C.: The Attitudes of Mothers of Male Schizophrenics Toward Child Behavior. *J. Abnorm. Soc. Psychol.*, 48:185, 1953.

50. Martin, M. G.: Examination of the Disturbed Child. *Current Medical Digest*, 27:57, 1960.

51. Mayo Clinic: *Clinical Examinations in Neurology*, 2nd Ed. Philadelphia, W. B. Saunders Co., 1963.

52. McConville, B. J. and Purohit, A. P.: Classifying Confusion: A study of results of inpatient treatment in a multidisciplinary children's center. *Amer. Jour. Orthopsychiatry*, 43, April, 1973.

53. Menninger, K.: *A Manual for Psychiatric Case Study.* New York, Grune & Stratton, Inc., 1952, pp. 98–107. 2nd Ed., 1962, pp. 85–99.

54. Menninger, K., Mayman, M. and Pruyser, P.: *The Vital Balance.* New York, Viking Press, 1963.

55. Merritt, H. H.: *A Textbook of Neurology*, 5th Ed. Philadelphia, Lea & Febiger, 1973.

56. Michigan Department of Mental Health: *The Michigan Picture Test.* Chicago, Science Research Associates, Inc., 1953.

57. Moustakas, C.: *Psychotherapy with Children.* New York, Harper & Brothers, 1959.

58. Nurnberger, J. I. and Hingtgen, J. N.: Is Symptom Substitution an Important Issue in Behavior Therapy. *Biological Psychiatry*, 7:221,1973.

59. Rabin, A. and Haworth, M. (Eds.): *Projective Techniques with Children.* New York, Grune & Stratton, 1960.

60. Ross, A.: *The Practice of Clinical Child Psychology.* New York, Grune & Stratton, 1959.

61. Rutter, M.: Classification and Categorization in Child Psychiatry. *J. Child Psychol. and Psychiat.*, 6:71, 1965.

62. Sabshin, M.: Psychiatric Perspectives on Normality. *Arch. Gen. Psychiat.*, 17:258–264, 1967.

63. Schwab, J. J. and Bronn, J.: Uses and Abuses of Psychiatric Consultation. *J.A.M.A.*, 205:65, 1968.

64. Sears, R. R., Macoby, E. E. and Levin, H.: *Patterns of Child Rearing.* Evanston, Row, Peterson and Co., 1957.

65. Shoben, E. J.: The assessment of Parental Attitudes in Relation to Child Adjustment. *Genetic Psychology Monographs.* 39: 101, 1949.

66. Silver, A. A.: Diagnostic Value of Three Drawing Tests for Children. *J. Pediat.* 37:129, 1950.

67. Simmons, J. E.: Interviewing, in *Ambulatory Pediatrics*, Green and Haggerty (Eds.). Philadelphia, W. B. Saunders Co., 1968.

68. Simmons, J. E., Ten Eyck, R., McNabb, R. C., Parr, M., Birch, B., and Coleman, B.: Parent Treatability, paper read at the Annual Meeting of AAPSC, Chicago, 1973.
69. Terman, L. and Merrill, M.: *Stanford-Binet Intelligence Scale.* 3rd Ed. Boston, Houghton Mifflin Co., 1960.
70. Tyler, E., Truumaa, A., and Henshaw, P.: Family Group Intake by a Child Guidance Clinic Team. *Arch. Gen. Psychiat.,* 6:214, 1962.
71. Wechsler, D.: *Manual for the Wechsler Preschool and Primary Scale of Intelligence.* New York, The Psychological Corporation, 1967.
72. ————: *Wechsler Intelligence Scale for Children.* New York, The Psychological Corporation, 1949.
73. Werkman, S. L.: The Psychiatric Diagnostic Interview with Children. *Amer. J. Orthopsychiatry.* 35:764, 1965.
74. Witmer, H. (Ed.): *Psychiatric Interviews with Children.* New York, The Commonwealth Fund, 1946.
75. Zuckerman, M. and Oltean, M.: Some Relationships Between Maternal Attitude Factors and Authoritarianism, Personality Needs, Psychopathology, and Self-acceptance. *Child Development,* 30:27, 1959.
76. Zuckerman, M., Barrett, B., Bragiel, R. M.: The Parental Attitudes of Parents of Child Guidance Cases. *Child Development,* 31:401, 1960.
77. Zuk, G. and Rubinstein, D.: A Review of Concepts in the Study and Treatment of Families of Schizophrenics; in *Intensive Family Therapy,* Boszormenyi-Nagy and Framo (Eds.). New York, Harper & Row, 1965, pp. 1–32.

Index

Affect: disturbances in, 91, 93, 98. *See also* Mood changes
Affectionless children, 45
Alpern Symptom Severity Rating Scale, 187-190, 193
American Board of Psychiatry and Neurology, Inc.: Child Psychiatry Subcommittee, 18
American Mental Hygiene Movement, 208
American Psychiatric Association Committee on Nomenclature and Statistics, 183
American Psychoanalytic Association, 20
Analysis of case data, 128
Anxiety: in interview, 1-2, 7, 9-10, 17-18; manifestations, 91; relief of, by medication, 223 sources, 38, 39-40. *See also* Separation anxiety
Attention span, 27-28
Autism, 79-87. *See also* Childhood schizophrenia

Behavior: acting out, 38, 43, 149; avoidance, 38-39, 84, 92; clinging, 5
meaning of, 11; normal age-appropriate, 79, 83; modification of, 224-225
problems of, 222
See also Separation anxiety
Bender Motor Gestalt Test, 175
Blake, William: on play, 22
Brain damage: compared with functional symptoms, 107

California Mental Maturity Test, 165
Central nervous system impairment, 125
Characterological disorders, 159
Child psychiatrist:
as consultant, 204-206, 207-209 and family resistance, 213-214 in pediatric teaching hospital, 209-210
psychiatric treatment by, 221-225
prejudices against, 206-207
relations of, with medical colleagues, 206-207
role of, in medical management, 216-217
selection of training candidates, 18-19, 211
as teacher. *See* Child psychiatrist, as consultant.
Child psychiatry:
origin of, 208
Childhood schizophrenia: case dynamics, 98; fantasies of, 44; prognosis, 111; semantic confusion, 87. *See also* Autism *and* Symbiotic psychosis
Chorea: hereditary (Huntington's), 100, 102
Classification system, 105-107; case with uncrystallized psychopathology, 190-192
ideal,
basis of, 181
necessity of, 192
purposes of, 181-182
types of, 180
versus formulation, 181

Colloquialisms, 21
Community psychiatry. *See* Consultation, and community psychiatry.
Confessions, 24
Conformity *vs.* nonconformity, 36
Conscience. *See* Superego
Constriction, 92
Consultant. *See* Child psychiatrist, as consultant.
Consultations: 202-226
  and community psychiatry, 204-205
  definition of, 203
  essential elements of, 210
  medical, 6-7
  in non-medical setting, 204-206
  in pediatric teaching hospital, 209-210
  process of, 211-213
  requests for,
    examples of, 211-212
    inappropriate, 211
  responsibility for, 202-203
  summary of, 225-226
  types of, 203-204, 225
Conversation: ability, 93; irrelevant, 90
Coordination: neuromuscular, 30, 42
Coping mechanisms, 38, 39, 84; pathological, 92
Counseling, 199, 218

Death: fears of, 31, 220
Defense mechanisms. *See* Coping mechanisms
Delinquent's resistance, 22
Denial. *See* Coping mechanisms
Dependency-deprived children, 45
Depression: maternal, 130, 133-134
  parental
    effects of, on child, 215-216
Developmental lag, 86
Diagnostic formulation, 124
  and child's environment, 191
    evaluation of, 193
  and nosological diagnosis, 180-193

"Diagnostic Synthesis": per Menninger, 109
Discipline: parental, 163
Doll play technique: structured, 157
Drawings, 45, 90, 155, 174
Draw-A-Person Test, 31, 100, 156-157
Dreams, 31, 45, 89, 90, 94, 155, 172
Drug therapy, 199
DSM-II, 180-181, 183-185, 192
  hazards of use of, 183-184
  and ICD-8, 183
Dynamic-genetic formulation: GAP Report #62, 109

Eclectic approach, 194
Educational lag, 195. *See also* School failure
Ego functions, 34-35, 79, 198; deviations, 111; regressions, 108; strength, 34
Enuresis, 150
Environment: influence of, on diagnosis, 191-192, 193
Etiology, 194, 198; mother-father-child interaction, 125
Evasion. *See* Coping mechanisms
Examiner: activity-passivity ratio, 7, 25; patient's distrust of, 12-13, 21
Expectation-reality discrepancy, 121

Family group interviews, 5, 116
Family group therapy, 199
Family resistance: consultant's ability to deal with, 213-214. *See also* Parental resistance
Fantasies: normal or abnormal, 37, 44, 93; in neurotic children, 43; sadistic, 44
Father: absence of, 149; passivity, 136-138, 169. *See also* Etiology
Fears, 88, 91, 96, 140, 142, 172, 173; examination of, 31; of being examined, 27, 92, 95; of death, 31

Formulation, 181
Free-association, 45
Friendships, 28, 95, 101

GAP #62, 180-181, 185-187
    symptom list
        special value of, 187
        use of, 189
    usefulness of, 192
Group therapy. *See* Family group
    therapy
Guilt: delinquent's, 23

Hallucinations, 30
Hallucinosis: acute, 221-222
    treatment of, 221-222
Handicaps: reaction of child to,
    222-223
Hansel and Gretel, 90, 93
Health: physical, 30
Hedonism, 43
Hospitalization: emergency
    psychiatric, 4
Huntington's chorea, 100, 102
Hypnosis: use of, to remove
    symptoms, 223-224

Identification, 28-29, 32, 47, 86,
    95; social, 36
Identity: psychosexual. *See*
    Identification
Idiographic study methods, 105
Illness: severity of, 79, 108, 125,
    194
Impulses: aggressive, 92; anti-
    social, 46; control of, 23, 38, 39,
    84; sexual, 92
Infantile autism. *See* Autism *and*
    Childhood schizophrenia
Intellectualization. *See* Coping
    mechanisms
Intelligence quotient: estimate of,
    47
International Classification of
    Disease (ICD-8), 183
Interrogation. *See* Interviewing
Interviewing: methods of, 6, 7, 9,
    17, 24-27; for research, 51.
    See also Family group interviews

Language ability: preschool, 85
Learning impairment, 97
Limit setting, 156, 163

Management: medical
        and psychiatric treatment,
        216-221
    role of child psychiatrist in,
        216-217
    psychiatric
        techniques in, 217-218
Mannerisms, 36
Marital relations, 131
Masturbation, 163
Medication: use of, to remove
    symptoms, 223
Memories: earliest, 31
Menstruation, 30
Mental status: children compared
    to adults, 16, 21
    examination of, 35-47, 80-102,
        212
Monsters, 172
Mood changes, 36, 83-84
Mother: relation with child, 99,
    125, 155, 156; relation with
    father, 168, 174; depression.
    See Depression, maternal
Motility, 42
Mourning, 12, 130-131

Narcissism, 47
Nervousness: child's concept of, 89
Neurological disease, 6-7
Nightmares. *See* Dreams
Nomenclature. *See* Classification
    system
Nomothetic study method, 105
Nonverbal children, 50-51
Normalcy, 20, 194, 197
Nosology: in adolescents, 99
    and diagnostic formulation,
        180-193

Object relations, 46
Obstinacy, 84
Onset of illness, 99
Orthopedic surgery, 126

Parent Treatability scale, 191
Parental adjustment, 114-115, 117, 150; child's view of, 29-30. *See* also Etiology
Parental resistance, 113, 118, 119, 120-121. *See also* Family resistance
Pathology: depth of, 44
Peer relations. *See* Friendships
Perception: apparatus, 37; pre-school child, 84-85
Physical health, 30
Play: meaning of, 12, 21-22, 26, 31, 39, 45
Playroom, 7
Premorbid adjustment, 99, 198
Prevention, 197
    primary, 205, 209
    secondary, 205, 209
Primary physician: psychological treatment by, 219-221
Primary process thinking, 21
Problems: child's view, 175; discussion of, 27, 42; revealed in play, 43, 44. *See also* Interviewing
Prognosis, 110-111, 195
Projection. *See* Coping mechanisms
Pseudomaturity, 89
Psychoanalysis: child, 20; theories, 108; training, 19-20
Psychological testing, 125
Psychopathogenesis. *See* Etiology
Psychosis: maternal, 162, 165-166; childhood. *See* Childhood schizophrenia
Psychotherapy, 16-17, 199

Questioning. *See* Interviewing

Racial prejudice, 154
Rationalization. *See* Coping mechanisms
Raven's Controlled Projection Test, 172
Reality contact, 30-31, 37
Recording: of interview, 34
Remissions: spontaneous, 200
Remedial education, 199

Reproduction: human. *See* Sex
Resistance, 21, 25, 88. *See also* Delinquent's resistance *and* Parental resistance
Right and wrong: sense of, 22-23, 32, 46, 101
Rorschach, 157-158

Schizoid child, 43
Schizophrenia: childhood type. *See* Childhood schizophrenia *and* Autism
School failure, 96, 97, 100, 161, 195
School phobia, 129, 184
Scoliosis, 151
Separation anxiety, 5, 139, 142. *See also* School phobia
Severity of illness, 79, 108, 125, 194
Sex: attitudes and knowledge, 23-24, 29, 38-39, 163
Sibling rivalry, 150
Silence: meaning of, 25. *See also* Resistance
Socioeconomic subculture. *See* Identification
Somatic symptoms, 30
Space relationships, 38
Speech: disturbances, 36; spontaneous, 42
Stanford Primary Achievement Test, 165
Stealing, 23
Stress, psychic, 218
Stress reaction, 86
Structured doll play technique, 157
Structured interviews for research, 51
Superego: examination of, 23; internalization of, 46, 86
Symbiotic psychosis (Mahler), 87
Symbolic play, 10-11, 17-18
Symptom: psychosomatic, 215. *See also* Alpern Symptom Severity Rating Scale
    removal of, 219, 223-225
        by hypnosis, 223-224
        by medication, 223

Symptom—*(Continued)*
  somatic
    in response to environmental
      stress, 215
Talents, 27-28
Techniques: psychiatric, 217-218
  use of, by family physician,
    217
Television, 89, 141
Thematic Apperception Test, 157
Therapy. *See* Treatment
Thinking: examination of, 27-28,
  42, 93; in preschool child, 85;
  tangential, 96
Third party payor:
  and classification system, 182
Three money bags, 31
Three wishes, 31, 45, 94, 141,
  155, 173
Tics, 36
Time relationships, 38
Toys. *See* Playroom
Treatment: case illustrations, 98,
    99, 143, 144-145, 160-161,
    175-176
  explanation of, to parents, 121;
  planning, 124, 126, 181, 199;
  psychiatric
    and medical management,
      216-221

Treatment: case illustrations—
(Continued)
    intensive
      identification of need for,
        213-214
      short term, 214-216
      therapeutic counseling in, 218
    psychological
      case illustrations of, 219-221,
        222, 223
      by consulting psychiatrist,
        221-225
      by primary physician, 219-221
Triage, 211

Unconscious phenomenon:
  observation of, 93
Uncooperativeness, 2-3, 6, 9-10

Value system, 46
Violence, 10-11, 101, 141
Vocabulary, 42
Vocational interests, 28-29

Wechsler Intelligence Scale for
  Children, 156, 158, 175
Wishes: examples, 43, 90, 91.
  See also Three wishes
Withdrawal, 41, 84